CONST
ITS CAUSI

CONSTIPATION:
ITS CAUSES AND CURE

Sri Swami Sivananda

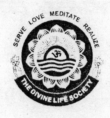

Published by

THE DIVINE LIFE SOCIETY

P.O. SHIVANANDANAGAR—249 192

Distt. Tehri-Garhwal, Uttaranchal, Himalayas, India

Price | **2006**   [**Rs. 60/-**

First Edition: 1956
Second Edition: 2002
Third Edition: 2006

[2,000 Copies]

ISBN 81-7052-189-0

ES 311

Published by Swami Vimalananda for
The Divine Life Society, Shivanandanagar, and printed by him
at the Yoga-Vedanta Forest Academy Press,
P.O. Shivanandanagar, Distt. Tehri-Garhwal, Uttaranchal,
Himalayas, India

SRI SWAMI SIVANANDA

Born on the 8th September, 1887, in the illustrious family of Sage Appayya Dikshitar and several other renowned saints and savants, Sri Swami Sivananda had a natural flair for a life devoted to the study and practice of Vedanta. Added to this was an inborn eagerness to serve all and an innate feeling of unity with all mankind.

His passion for service drew him to the medical career; and soon he gravitated to where he thought that his service was most needed. Malaya claimed him. He had earlier been editing a health journal and wrote extensively on health problems. He discovered that people needed right knowledge most of all; dissemination of that knowledge he espoused as his own mission.

It was divine dispensation and the blessing of God upon mankind that the doctor of body and mind renounced his career and took to a life of renunciation to qualify for ministering to the soul of man. He settled down at Rishikesh in 1924, practised intense austerities and shone as a great Yogi, saint, sage and Jivanmukta.

In 1932 Swami Sivananda started the Sivanandashram. In 1936 was born The Divine Life Society. In 1948 the Yoga-Vedanta Forest Academy was organised. Dissemination of spiritual knowledge and training of people in Yoga and Vedanta were their aim and object. In 1950 Swamiji undertook a lightning tour of India and Ceylon. In 1953 Swamiji convened a 'World Parliament of Religions'. Swamiji is the author of over 300 volumes and has disciples all over the world, belonging to all nationalities, religions and creeds. To read Swamiji's works is to drink at the Fountain of Wisdom Supreme. On 14th July, 1963 Swamiji entered Mahasamadhi.

CONTENTS

CONSTIPATION:

ITS CAUSES AND CURE

Chapter I
PRAYERS

Maha Mrityunjaya Mantra

ॐ त्र्यंबकं यजामहे सुगन्धि पुष्टिवर्धनम् ।
उर्वारुकमिवबन्धनान्मृत्योर्मुक्षीय मामृतात् ॥

Om Tryambakam yajamahe
Sugandhim pushti vardhanam
Urvaarukamiva bandhanaan
Mrityormuksheeya maamritat

Meaning

We worship the three-eyed One (Lord Siva) who is fragrant and who nourishes well all beings; may He liberate us from death for the sake of Immortality even as the cucumber is severed from its bondage (to the creeper).

Benefits

1. This Maha Mrityunjaya Mantra is a life-giving Mantra. In these days, when life is very complex and accidents are an everyday affair, this Mantra wards off deaths by snake-bite, lightning, motor-accidents, fire-accidents, cycle-accidents, water-accidents, air-accidents and accidents of all descriptions. Besides, it has a great curative effect. Again, diseases pronounced incurable by doctors are cured by this Mantra, when chanted with sincerity, faith and devotion. It is a weapon against all diseases. It is a Mantra to conquer death.

2. It is also a Moksha Mantra. It is Lord Siva's Mantra. It bestows long life (Deergha Ayush), peace (Shanti), wealth

(Aisvarya), prosperity (Pushti), satisfaction (Tushti) and Immortality (Moksha).

3. On your birthday, repeat one lakh of this Mantra or at least 50,000; perform Havan and feed Sadhus, the poor and the sick. This will bestow on you long life, peace and prosperity.

4. Kindly consecrate one Maala or more daily to Sri Swami Sivanandaji!

Hari Om Tat Sat

Prayer for Health

O adorable Lord of ocean of compassion,
Salutations and prostrations unto Thee.
OM Namah Sivaya.
OM Namo Narayanaya.
OM Namo Bhagavate Vaasudevaya.
O Lord, grant me good health and strength,
Free me from constipation and all other diseases.
Without good health and strength
I cannot practise concentration,
I cannot do any kind of Sadhana.
Thou art my sole refuge,
Thou art my father, mother, friend and preceptor.
I am Thine, all is Thine,
Thy Will be done, O Lord.

Antaryamin Upanishad

He who dwells within this constipation,
He who is within this constipation,
But whom constipation does not know,
Whose body constipation is,
Who rules constipation from within,
Is thy Inner Ruler, Immortal,
Antaryamin, Amritam,

Know Him, realise Him,
And be free from constipation, body and death.

Thus Spoke Constipation

I alone cause intestinal colic,
Piles, Varicocele, and auto-intoxication.
I produce fever, depression, headache,
Lassitude, lack of concentration, vertigo,
General ill-health, boils, acne, anaemia,
Palpitation, nocturnal emissions.
I establish drug habit, enema habit,
I assume various forms, Acute, Chronic, habitual
and occasional.
I make the tongue furred, appetite poor.
I cause much straining at stools,
And diarrhoea from irritation of scybalae.

All Medical Systems Are Necessary

Maya is plurality.
Minds are different.
Temperaments are diverse.
Constituents are different.
Hence different systems of medicine are needed.
Allopathy suits some;
Homeopathy suits others.
Senna is agreeable to some,
While cascara is suitable to others.
Behold God in everything.
See God in everything.
Learn to become wise.
Do not fight and quarrel.

Weights and Measures

1. Weight for Solids

1 drachm	60 grains
8 drachms	1 ounce

1 ounce	437.5 grains
1 pound	16 oz., 7000 grains
20 grains	1 scrupple
180 grains	1 tola or 1 rupee weight
5 and ⅝ lb. Av.	1 seer
3 lbs 2 oz Av.	1 viss
3 lbs 9 oz Tro.	1 viss

2. Measure for Fluids

1 minim	more or less one drop
60 minims	1 drachm
8 drachms	1 ounce
20 ounces	1 pint
8 pints	1 gallon
Quart	2 pints
Teaspoonful	1 drachm
Dessert spoonful	2 drachms
Table spoonful	4 drachms
Wine glassful	2½ ounces

3. Weights and Measures

32 kunrumanis (gunjas)	= 1 varahanidai
9 panavidai	= 1 varahanidai
1 palam	= 10 varahanidais
1 kazhanji	= 1¼ varahanidai
1 tola	= 3¼ varahanidais
50 palams	= 1 thooku
1 panavidai	= 3 kunrumanis
approximately	edai or 5 grains
16 salli edai	= 1 palam
5 seers of liquid (volume)	= 1 Madras measure
1 seer (volume – above)	= 40 ounces of water

Chapter II

CONSTIPATION

Introduction

Constipation is otherwise known by the names *faecal accumulation, costive bowels.* It is more common among women than men and is even natural to some persons. It may be occasional or habitual.

The human body may safely be compared to a municipal town. The intestines or entrails or bowels of the human frame exactly represent municipal carts which remove the solid refuse from a town. A person suffering from constipation can no more be healthy than can a town whose street sweepings, excreta, kitchen waste, house waste, stable waste, factory waste, etc., are not got rid off. Accumulation of faecal matter proves deleterious to health, and constipation of a long-standing nature exerts as bad an effect on the health of a man as accumulation of refuse matter in a town has on the health of the community at large.

The action of the bowels is to a large extent a question of habit. The bowels should be moved at least once daily. Some persons answer the calls of nature once, or twice daily, while in some, movement of the bowels occurs once every two or three days without any appreciable ill-effect upon the general health, and unattended by unpleasant symptoms.

Proper elimination is almost as important as a correct diet. Even when the right food is eaten, good health will not be enjoyed unless waste matter is properly removed from the system. Faulty elimination is an exceedingly common condition today owing to faulty habits of eating and living. Inactivity of the liver and kidneys is often associated with this complaint.

Dangers of Constipation

Though constipation is regarded as a trifling ailment, its phase of grave import must not be ignored. With its usual train of attendant evils as nausea or a tendency to vomit, loathing for food which amounts to even anorexia or loss of appetite, griping pains in abdomen, a feeling of discomfort and depression, etc., constipation predisposes to a host of ailments as piles, prolapse of rectum or anus, poisoning of the system, etc. There seems reason to believe that some people's intestines are weak from birth. This is not surprising as it is well-known that weakness in other organs, such as the heart and stomach, may be passed on from parent to child. This is not a haphazard trick on the part of Nature, but the simple working out of the law of cause and effect, bad habits of the parents having their effect upon the lives of their offspring.

Constipation is often the frequent result of sluggish action of the bowels induced by sedentary habits and avocations, lack of exercises, general debility, senile decay or degeneracy, habitual neglect of calls of nature, errors in diet. The diet of the modern civilised races is too concentrated and too rich in protein and sugar. Consequently the intestine does not contain enough waste matter to stimulate it into action. In a natural diet containing a good proportion of wholemeal bread, fresh fruit, and vegetables, this difficulty is overcome.

Health of the Bowel

The health of the bowel is of paramount importance.

The general health of the individual largely depends upon the health of the bowels. The digestive processes in the intestines should be kept up properly. The faecal matter should not accumulate in the bowels. If it accumulates decomposition and fermentation will take place. There will be formation of foul gases. The poisonous or toxic products of decomposition will be absorbed and autointoxication or faecal toxaemia will take place and there will be various unpleasant symptoms and deterioration of health.

You should have a very clear broad motion daily in the early morning. This is a sign of bowel-health and general good health. A stagnant bowel is a centre of diseases. The bowel must be kept as clean as possible.

Vegetables green and leafy, fruits, milk, diet rich in organic salts and cellulose or roughage keep the bowel healthy and efficient.

Myrobalan, Indian Gooseberry (Amala) Bael leaves, Bael fruit, lemon, bland, non-irritating foods etc., tone the bowels and ensure bowel-health.

Too much Chutney, pickles, spices, condiments, chillies, too much tamarind and other irritating foods, liquors spoil the bowel-health.

The stools of the chief meal of the day should pass out of the body next day. If this is done the health of the bowel and the general health will be surely maintained.

If there is accumulation of faecal matter, take an enema.

Have abdominal massage. This will ensure good bowel-health.

A healthy bowel means a healthy brain, a healthy in and a healthy heart too.

The Small and Large Intestines

The small intestine extends from the stomach above to the large intestine below. It is a convoluted tube about 20 feet in length. It fills the greater part of the front abdominal cavity. Its diameter is about 2 inches at the beginning. It gradually diminishes in size and is hardly an inch in diameter at its lower end. It is divided into 3 portions viz., the duodenum, the jejunum and the ileum.

The duodenum is twelve finger's breadth in length. The jejunum is 7½ feet in length. The ileum constitutes the balance of the small intestine.

The large intestine is about 5 feet long and from two and a half to one and a half inches wide. It extends from the ileum to the anus. It is divided into three parts, viz., the caecum with the vermiform appendix; colon and rectum.

The colon is subdivided into the ascending, transverse and descending colon with the sigmoid flexure. The rectum is from 6 to 8 inches long. The anal opening is guarded by two circular muscles, the internal and external sphincters.

What Is Peristalsis?

The alternate contractions and dilatations of adjoining segments of the intestines or bowels is termed peristalsis. It produces a wave-like motion or vermicular movement (worm-like) along the intestinal tract. Have you seen the movement of the caterpillar? Peristalsis is similar to the movement.

When food is taken, it is thrust into the oesophagus or gullet by the action of the pharynx. The muscular wall of the oesophagus just above the bolus contracts and pushes it down into the next lower part. Then the wall of the part contracts and pushes the mass a little further down and so on. In this way the food is finally thrust into the stomach by a series of contractions of each part of the oesophagus in succession. This is also spoken of as peristaltic action.

Drink also is taken in exactly the same way as food. It does not fall down the pharynx and gullet, but each gulp is grasped and passed down.

The muscular coat of the small intestines is made up of two layers, an outer longitudinal, an inner circular. The circular fibres of any part are able to contract successively in such a manner, that the upper fibres or those nearer the stomach, contact before the lower ones, or those nearer the large intestine. The contents of the intestines are constantly being propelled by successive and progressive narrowing of their calibre (peristaltic movement), from their upper towards their lower parts. The same peristaltic movement takes place in the large intestine from the ileo-caecal valve to the anus or the termination of the alimentary canal.

Defective peristalsis is due to atony or loss of tone of the muscular coat of the intestines, old age, anaemia. Atony of the colon causes constipation. If the intestine are toned by the practice of Asanas, Pranayama or abdominal massage, constipation will be cured.

Faeces and Defaecation

By the abstraction of all the soluble constituents and especially by the withdrawal of water, the liquid contents become, as they approach the rectum, changed into a firm and solid mass of waste matter, ready for ejection from the body and called faeces.

The faeces consists of the undigested and indigestible substances of the food. Among them are the elastic fibres of connective tissue, the callulose, which is the chief constituent of the envelopes encasing the cells of plants, and the indigestible mucin of mucus. These three materials, together with some water, some undigested food-stuffs and some excretory substances found in the various secretions poured into the alimentary canal, form the bulk of the material expelled from the body.

The normal rate of passage through the intestine is from the ingestion of food to the caecum 4½ hours, hepatic flexure 6½ hours, splenic flexure 9 hours; entering the pelvic colon at 12 hours; and rectum at 18 hours.

The average daily amount of faeces in health is 120-180 grm. (about 4 ounces).

The colour of normal faeces is partly due to stercobilin, partly to chlorophyll and other pigments.

The odour of the faeces is due to the presence of indol and skatol.

In obstinate constipation the form and consistence of the stools may be such drier and harder than normal, and even friable. The stools of constipation have often the form of round balls, frequently coated with mucus.

II

Defaecation is the term applied to the act of expelling the faeces from the rectum.

(a) The food taken into the mouth and masticated is mixed with saliva and swallowed undergoes gastric digestion in the stomach; passes into the intestines, and is subjected to the action of the secretions of the liver and pancreas, with which it there becomes mixed and finally after the more or less complete extraction of the nutritive constituents, the residue mixed up with certain secretions of the intestines, leaves the body as the faeces.

By the time, the contents of the intestines have reached the ileo caecal valve, a great deal of the nutritious matter has bean removed. Still even in the large intestine, some nutritious matter has still to be acted upon.

In the caecum and commencement of the large intestine, changes are taking place, apparently somewhat of fermentation, whereby the contents become acid.

(b) Defaecation is a reflex action carried out by the spinal cord as soon as it has been started by the will. The sensory surface is the mucous membrane of the rectum, the necessary stimulus is supplied as the result of the distention of rectum by the accumulated faeces.

Chapter III

CAUSES OF CONSTIPATION

Constipation is insufficient action of the bowels, delay in the passage of the contents of the bowels, causing hard, dry faeces Scybala. The delay is usually in the pelvic colon or the rectum. A useful and simple test consists in giving a tablespoonful of powdered charcoal at night. It should normally have completely disappeared from the stools before 48 hours.

To ensure the due evacuation of the bowels the digestive functions of the stomach and small intestine and the secretion of bile and pancreatic juice must all be in proper working order. The colon must absorb some of the water from the fluid faeces, rendering them of a proper consistency for expulsion. The intestinal muscles must be in a healthy condition. Therefore constipation may be caused by interference with any of these functions and hence may be due to large variety of causes.

The retention of hard stools may give rise to an alternating diarrhoea, which leads to error in diagnosis. Piles result from habitual constipation.

The Chief Causes Are:

1. **Causes which produce stony or loss of tone of the muscles of the intestines:** (a) general diseases such as anaemia or poverty of blood, the specific fevers, chronic Bright's disease (of the kidney), (b) nervous diseases, such as nervous debility, paraplegia (c) sedentary habits.

2. **Errors of Diet:** A diet which does not sufficiently stimulate the bowel. There may not be enough food (too

little or poor food, deficiency of vitamins), or it may be too dry (deficient fluid ingesta) or it may not cause sufficient mechanical irritation (defect of vegetable matters, — no vegetables, no food, with coarse residue). The faeces may become dry through loss of water by other channels, diabetes, granular kidney, vomiting, perspiration.

3. **Causes of Defective Peristalsis:** (a) Sedentary habits, (b) depressing emotions, anxiety, worry, etc., cause sympathetic inhibition, hence spasm, (c) old age and other conditions with poor general tone, such as anaemia, (d) prolonged disregard of the calls of nature with dilatation of rectum and pelvic colon, consequent on blunted sensation, (e) weak abdominal muscles, (f) atony or loss of tone of the colon, (g) some febrile states, (h) endocrine disorder, specially deficient acting of thyroid and pituitary, (i) reflex spasm as in catarrh of the colon or disease of the womb, (j) diseases of the brain or spinal cord, such as tabes, and cerebral tumour.

4. **Deficiency of bile or intestinal secretions:** (a) Functional inactivity of the liver, (b) profuse vomiting, (c) excessive loss of fluid by skin or kidneys, (d) astringents, such as chalk or catechu. Hard waters also act in this way.

5. Mechanical obstructions such as 'Kinks '.

6. Neglect of the daily call to defaecation. This leads gradually to extinction of the impulse.

7. Inhibition of the reflex action of the bowel. On account of painful defaecation or abdominal pain.

In one type the delay may be in the colon. There is slow passage through the intestines to the rectum. In another type there is delay and difficulty in emptying the rectum ("dyschezia"). The rectum is constantly full of hardened faeces. It may become blocked by scybalous masses. The passage to the pelvic colon is at a normal rate.

Pressure of the faecal matter on the intrapelvic veins may cause haemorroids or varicocele. Where the lower bowel is much loaded, there may be pressure on the lumbar or sacrel nerves and pain down the back or part of the left thigh.

Another common cause of sluggishness in the bowels is lack of fluid. In the large intestine water is normally absorbed from the faecal mass and thus it is rendered too hard if insufficient water be present.

The wearing of tight belts, tight girdles, rigid corsets and waist bands impedes the free and natural movements of the abdomen and induces constipation.

Country people hardly suffer from costiveness of the bowels and it is only in the case of the people of urban localities whose artificial mode of life forces than even to the putting off answering the calls, that constipation is frequently met with. This failure to heed the calls of nature is another important cause of constipation. Neglect in this respect is much more common than might be supposed, and frequently it can be proved to be the starting point of constipation. Therefore it is most important to have what may be termed 'habit time'. This means that a regular time should be fixed each day for defaecation, and an attempt should be made to empty the bowels even if no desire is felt.

Constipation in babies is due to improper feeding either of the child or mother. Condensed milk binds the bowels and this difficulty may be obviated by having recourse to fresh cow's milk. Constipation occurs from sluggish action of either liver or small bowels or large intestines. Failure to answer the calls in time causes undue dryness of the faecal matter by the absorption of a portion of water and constipation results.

Crusade Against Constipation

Delay in the passage of faeces through the intestines or delay in their evacuation is constipation. Disturbance of the digestive system most commonly manifests itself in the form of constipation or diarrhoea. If food taken does not pass out within twenty-four hours, it is a slow action of the intestines or bowels. It is constipation if it does not pass off within forty-eight hours. Whereas a quick passage of food through the bowel is called diarrhoea. Diarrhoea may be a symptom of constipation. The accumulated faecal matter irritates the lower bowel and causes diarrhoea.

Constipation may be a symptom of certain acute diseases such as typhoid fever or of chronic diseases such as affections of the liver or stomach or of anaemia or poverty of blood. Or it may be due to mechanical obstruction of some part of the bowel.

There are three varieties of constipation. (1) Intestinal constipation: there is delay in the passage of the stools through the intestines, usually in the colon. (2) Rectal Constipation: here the intestinal transit time is normal but the motions accumulate in the pelvic colon and rectum. (3) Greedy colon: here excessive absorption reduces the bulk of the stools.

One kind of constipation is usually due to an accumulation of faecal matter in the rectum which becomes insensitive to the stimulus of distension. It is not due to delay in the emptying of the colon. If you give large doses of purgatives in this type of constipation there will be increase in the toxic absorption from the bowels.

The contents will become liquid and the food will be hurried into its lower reaches where fermentation takes place.

The delay in the passage of the faeces through the

intestines may be due to the small bulk of the stools on account of insufficient food. It may be due also to a diet poor in residue such as callulose, to insufficient fluid contents, to excessive loss of fluid as in diabetes, to excessive sweating or to excessive absorption as in greedy colon.

It may also be due to a large bulk of stools as in gluttons, which causes difficulty in propulsion, to weakness of the intestinal walls, to obstruction by growth in the intestines, by intussuesception and to loss of muscle tone.

Ordinarily the bowels should be moved ones daily, but to some this does not naturally occur. Hence there are unpleasant symptoms as giddiness, heaviness in the bowels, etc. For constipation of this kind, medicines as a rule, are not necessary. Exercise, more fluid and fruit diet will remove the evil.

The barium meal will indicate where the delay takes place. Normally the meal should reach the caecum in 5 hours, the hepatic flexure in 7 hours, the splenic flexure in 9 hours, the pelvic colon in 12 hours and the rectum in 18 hours.

Faecal Toxaemia: If the faeces accumulates in the bowels, they ferment and decompose after some time. Various kinds of toxins or poisons are formed in the bowel. They are slowly absorbed into the blood and cause a kind of toxaemia or slow blood poising. This is called faecal toxaemia. The symptom and sign of faecal toxaemia are lassitude, fever, mental depression, lack of appetite, furred tongue, headache, a sallow complexion with loss of flesh, nervous debility, anorexia or loss of appetite, flatulence, abdominal discomfort or colic.

There are some doctors who trace the origin of all diseases to constipation, just as there are some doctors who trace the origin of all diseases to pyorrhoea, stomach or blood. But the real cause is Prarabdha or Karma. Vedantins trace the cause of all diseases to the mind (Vasanas and cravings), Adi Vyadhi. According to Vedantins and Raja Yogins the primary causes are bad thoughts If these thoughts are destroyed, all bodily diseases will vanish.

Hard stools are due to costive condition of the bowels. If the stools are hard know that more water has been extracted from them than is necessary. The faeces stay in the bowels for a longer time and so water is lost. Drink more water. The faeces will become very soft.

If the bowels are sluggish in expelling the faeces, drinking of abundant water will not remove the hard lumps. In such cases enema will bring the desired effect. The bowels must be washed out.

There must be abundant roughage in the food-stuff. Take more of leafy and fibrous matter and husk of cereals. These will give bulk to the faecal matter. You will get soft motion.

Correct the condition without the use of purgatives. Take recourse to natural methods. Some drugs irritate the bowels, cause the contents to become fluid, increase the toxic absorption and lessen the response of the bowel to natural stimuli. Thus the condition is rendered worse.

Do not neglect the desire to answer the calls. Fix a special time for answering the calls (morning 4 or 5 a.m.) and stick to it. Even if there is no desire to defaecate, make the attempt at the proper time. Do not make hurried visits. Wait till there is complete evacuation.

Do not bother if there is no evacuation in a day. Do not worry. Do not be anxious. This anxiety will upset the nervous mechanism of bowel evacuation and will encourage the use of purgatives.

Take plenty of water. Take fruits and vegetables. Take sufficient quantity of food. Take a tumbler of water as soon as you get up from the bed. These supply the bulk which is necessary to stimulate the bowels to pass its contents along.

See that the bulk of the food is sufficient. Constipation is due to insufficient quantity and unsuitable quality of food.

Excessive absorption of fluid from the colon is also the cause for constipation. In this case drink much larger quantity of fluid.

Spend sufficient time in answering the calls of nature. The bad act of rushing the act is often contracted at school.

A tendency to constipation is natural to many persons, especially to women. Regulate the system in such a way that there is neither constipation nor diarrhoea. Then alone you will keep good health.

Observe the rules of health and hygiene. Take proper, wholesome food and drink in moderation. Be regular in your exercise, Kirtan, meditation, Asanas and Pranayama. You will be free from constipation and diarrhoea.

Massage the abdomen nicely. This may assist defaecation. Start from the right lower corner across the top of the abdomen and down the left side to the left lower corner. Use gingely or mustard oil for massage.

A teaspoonful of liquid extract of Cascara Sagrada or Cascara Evacuant is very useful.

If all these measures fail, a small enema or a glycerine suppository may be found very effective in cases where there is accumulation of faecal matter in the rectum. It can be tried in the early morning at the time the bowels are required to open.

For temporary constipation, castor oil, mercurials, salines, compounds of sulphur and senna, rhubarb or cascara are prescribed.

For chronic constipation, a small morning dose of sulphate of magnesia, anthracenes, vegetable laxatives or liquid paraffin usually with agar-agar are given at bed time.

Constipation with anaemia and amernorrhoea is often treated with aloes and ferrous-sulphate.

Purgatives are to be *given with caution* in suspected intestinal obstruction, intestinal haemorrhage, pregnancy, menorrhagia and in severe asthenia and also in enteric and eruptive fevers and in kala-azar.

Chapter IV

HINTS ON TREATMENT OF CONSTIPATION

1. The accumulation of stools in the bowels causes great pressure on the various abdominal organs and upsets normal condition of nerves. Therefore eradicate constipation.

2. The accumulation of faeces in the rectum causes pressure on the blood vessels and this gives rise to bleeding piles or haemorrhoids. Hence, nip constipation in its bud.

3. Fruits like mangoes, bael, papaya are highly beneficial in curing constipation.

4. Starchy food may be partially replaced by fruits.

5. Massage is a potent helper in curing constipation.

6. Some do not experience any bad symptom even if the bowels only move every other day or the third day.

7. One may not be constipated although the bowels only move every other day.

8. Chronic constipation is a common complaint which often causes no symptoms. The bowels may be opened daily, but evacuation is incomplete. The patient is not conscious that he has constipation.

9. Normally the bowel should be emptied up to the splenic flexure.

10. Occasional constipation may be removed by the use of a dose of castor oil, 1 or 2 ounces, or myrobalan or a dose of Enos' Fruit Salt.

11. Habitual constipation is usually accompanied by loss of appetite, furred tongue, bad taste in the mouth, indigestion, flatulence or wind in the bowels, difficult breathing, malnutrition, anaemia or poverty of blood, headache, flushing of the face, sores in the mouth, irritability of temper, disturbed sleep, etc.

12. Porridge, stewed prunes, brown wholemeal bread, carrots, stewed fruits, fruit pudding, butter, cabbage, cauliflower, beans, brussels sprouts are all beneficial in constipation.

13. If the faeces are very hard they may be softened by injecting with a syringe 4 ounces of warm olive oil into the rectum at night.

14. Infusion of senna pods is highly beneficial. Allow the pods to remain in cold water for 24 hours.

15. A combination of liquid Paraffin and cascara is very effective.

16. Prolonged use of artificially digested foods causes constipation. Too dry a diet also produces costiveness of bowels.

17. The contents of the bowels must be semisolid, non-irritating and free from undigested food. Then alone the colon will work efficiently in inducing good peristalsis.

18. If you reduce your diet all at once, it will produce a temporary constipation.

19. Asanas can remove constipation only if it is due to atonic condition of the nerves and muscles, and walls of the intestines. If it is due to insufficiency of food, they cannot cure this kind of constipation.

20. Rectum should be emptied by giving a dose of an ounce of castor oil. Castor oil acts in three hours. Castor oil should be followed by an enema. This will produce an

immediate cleaning. By the action of castor oil there will be removal of debris from up also.

It is a fashion nowadays to blame every illness on the poor old colon and the fear of terrible consequences due to constipation. Most of them never happen at all. Merely use of commonsense in regulating the digestion will relieve many of the troubles.

The term such as auto-intoxication, colonic stagnation are not having much importance. Repeated irritation of the colon by laxative is not advisable. You must treat the colon very kindly.

Unless it is advised by the doctor, cathartics should not be used. People are becoming increasingly alive to the cathartic danger in its relation to appendicitis. During any inflammation of the intestine, it can spread throughout the abdomen to cause deadly peritonitis.

The causes that produce constipation must be ascertained and the aim of the treatment should be directed towards the eradication of the cause. It is only by the discovery and appreciation of the causes that are in operation that constipation may safely be combated. In some cases medicines prove worse than useless; purgatives of every description do more harm than good. Discretion, commonsense and sound judgment certainly go a long way in the treatment of constipation as in the cure of other diseases.

Most cases of constipation can be cured by rational methods without the use of drugs. In the first place, all causes which lead to the condition must be avoided. If the patient has led a sedentary life, he must see that he gets the necessary exercise, by walking or riding, or by artificial means such as kneading the abdomen.

The cultivation of the habit of regular defaecation is of

paramount importance. One should go to the closet every day at a fixed hour in the early morning whether the effort is successful or not and by such systematic solicitation his endeavour, will certainly be crowned with success. Hurried visits to the latrines and imperfect answering the calls should be deprecated. Sedentary habit must be avoided and plenty of exercise must be taken in the open air. Fruits, fresh vegetables, cabbages, relieve the costiveness and effect softened motions in the morning. A cup of hot coffee acts as a prompt laxative. Measures should be taken to nip the constipation of an occasional nature in its bud lest become habitual. It is only when these auxiliary measures fail to produce the desired effect that we must resort to medical agents. In this connection it will not be out of place to mention the varieties of *aperients* and their action.

There have never been as many aperients to choose from as at the present day, and no difficulty should be experienced in selecting something suitable for one's particular needs. In order to assist in this, we may say a few words about some of the common laxatives in use today.

Purgatives may be divided into the following classes: laxatives, simple purgatives, and saline purgatives. Laxatives are substances which slightly increase the action on the bowels by stimulating the intestinal muscle. Examples of this class are the following: wholemeal bread, most fruits, treacle, honey, sulphur, cassia, olive and castor oil, liquid paraffin, etc.

Cathartics, aperients or purgatives increase or expedite the evacuation of the intestines. Laxatives as sulphur, figs, olive oil, prunes, etc., produce only softened motions, by simply quickening the movements of the bowels, while drastic purgatives as jalap, colocynth bowels violently.

Epsom salt (magnesium sulphate) and Glauber's salt (sodium sulphate) are termed saline purgatives. Cholagogue purgatives act upon the liver, increase the secretion of bile and produce greenish liquid motions. Under this head may be mentioned, calomel, podophyllin, Euonymin, etc.

Saline purgatives act by drawing fluid from the tissues into the intestine, thus stimulating it to action. Magnesium sulphate, or Epsom salt, is perhaps the best known in this class. Other examples are potassium tartrate, sodium tartrate, potassium acid tartrate, potassium sulphite. Too much cannot be said about the value of fruits as laxatives. Take the fig for an example. Its value as an aid in intestinal troubles has long been known. Now comes a new discovery by science that there is added to its laxative qualities an enzyme which has remarkable powers in the destruction of intestinal parasites. Thus the natural remedies do more, rather than less, than what is expected of them. Also, it has been noted that fruits, when eaten in season are well suited to those bowel disorders which tend to be seasonal – they are timed for digestive disturbances.

Practical Hints on Diet

The diet must receive careful attention. Little or no flesh-food should be eaten. If the stomach is healthy, coarse food should be taken to produce roughage for the intestine to act upon. The diet should contain a large proportion of fresh foods such as lettuce, celery, tomatoes, and vegetables. Fruits are of the first importance. Prunes, figs, oranges, apples, and cooked fruits should be eaten freely, especially at breakfast time. Soft foods such as white bread, tea cakes, pastry, and all rich foods are not good. Water should be drunk freely on rising and between meals.

By attending to these points it should be possible to cure

most cases of constipation without the use of drugs or the enema.

Where there is a tendency to constipation, the diet should contain a liberal supply of fruits and anything in the laxative class may be tried. Many of these are domestic remedies. In almost every case the diet will be found to be at fault, and if this be corrected and proper exercises taken, a cure will usually result.

Food Allowed in Cases of Constipation

Choose the coarser breads with bran or wholemeal when possible. The bread should be taken in fairly large quantities and the kinds varied from time to time. It should never be new. The crust also should be eaten. Toast with plenty of butter is good. Nuts are usually contraindicated but in some cases dry walnuts or Brazil nuts well masticated appear to help. Oatmeal, crushed oats with sugar and milk or golden syrup, or old fashioned treacle; cabbages, salads with abundant oil, apples, figs, prunes, dates, oranges, grapes, bananas, straw berries, currents, etc.; jam, preserved fruits; hot or cold water; tea always freshly made and never strong are taken with meat. Coffee, thin cocoa, waters as Carlsbad, Kapler malt extract and Depler solution.

Foods Forbidden In Cases of Constipation

New bread and pastry; eggs, peas, new potatoes, tapioca, nuts of all kinds.

General Directions

1. Insist upon the patient taking a full quantity of fluid, for an adult at least two and a half to three pints daily. Many women suffering from constipation will be found to take only one to one and a quarter pints daily. Their constipation often depends upon this alone and yields when sufficient quantity of liquid is taken.

2. This fluid may well include a tumblerful of water, cold or hot, *immediately* on getting out of bed in the morning, and a tumblerful of hot water at bed time. Where hot water, with or without a saline aperient is ordered to be taken in the morning the effect is often enhanced if it be slowly sipped while dressing.

3. Absolutely forbid taking meat with tea; insist upon fruit or jam, or honey or treacle with farinaceous foods and order every night early morning a full quantity of such fruit as stewed figs, baked apples, bananas, etc.

4. The body should be warmly clothed to avoid the skin getting chilled and the feet kept warm and try by thick boots, with a cork or asbestos cloth.

5. Abdominal massage for ten minutes before rising, every morning. This (which can readily be done by the patient), followed by the cold or hot water on rising is often sufficient to produce a speedy evacuation.

6. Regular exercise, especially of those kinds which bring the abdominal muscles into play.

7. Insist upon the habit on regular hour every morning for the bowels to act, whether there be desire or not.

Drugs

The majority of cases can be cured without drugs if the proper treatment is begun sufficiently early. Every method should be tried before drugs are used to relieve constipation.

Vichy water drunk freely is very safe and helpful. Carlsbad salts may be taken in a tumbler of hot water as the first thing in the morning with great advantage. Half to one teaspoonful of Liquid Extract of Cascara may be taken at bed time.

In constipation of infant, glycerin may be injected into the bowels or a pointed bit of soap may be inserted in the anus. A few drops of castor oil is a safest remedy to be given to a newly born infant if the bowels are constipated,

Stewed figs eaten freely are an excellent laxative and a baked apple at bed time will also do immense good.

If the above measures fail, take 2 teaspoonfuls of magnesium Sulphite or Sodium Sulphate or Eno's Fruit Salt in the morning in 4 ounces of water. Drink a tumblerful of water later on.

Liquid Paraffin can be taken at night. The dose is from two teaspoonfuls to one tablespoonful. Petrolagar or Agarol are highly beneficial.

Chapter V

LAXATIVES AND PURGATIVES

Individuals have idiosyncrasies (peculiarities) of constitution about laxative action of different articles of diet. There are articles of diet of which the individual may have experienced of having laxative action upon him. Such articles should be taken along with food.

Cathartic: A drug that promotes evacuation from the bowels. It is divided into (1) laxative which induces gentle bowel movement. Example: Figs, prunes, phenolphthalein, etc. (2) purgative which produces copious, repeated and more watery motions. Example: Pulvis, Jalap, etc.

Cholagogue (Pitthakari): A remedy that promotes the secretion or excretion of bile. Example. Podophyllin, calomel, euonymir, walnut seed, etc.

Hydragogue (Jalavirochani): A drug that produces watery motions by inducing free secretion from the intestinal glands and removing much serum from the intestinal blood vessels. Example: Croton. This is a very drastic purgative.

Laxative (Malakari): A remedy that loosens the bowels, a milk purgative. Example. Walnut seed, liquorice, fig, castor oil, linseed, potatoes, sesamum, Bengal-gram, sugarcane, grapes, amalaka, myrobalan, papaya, tamarind fruit, asafoetida, radish, plantain fruit, bael fruit, methi leaves, ground-nut.

Purgative (Virochani): A remedy that causes copious watery evacuation of the bowels. Example: Castor oil, Jalap, etc.

Salines are purgatives which produce watery motion, e.g., Epsom Salt, (magnesium sulphate), and Glauber's Salt (sodium sulphate).

Laxatives
(Allopathic Patent Medicines)

1. California Syrup of Figs (Calfig). 2. Cascara Evacuvent. 3. Castophine. 4. Laxcasto. 5. Brooklax. 6. Bonamint — Chewing-gum Laxative. 7. Feenament — Chewing-gum Laxative. 8. Becham's Pills. 9. Bile Beans. 10. Carter's Little Liver pills. 11. Purgen. 12. Purgoids (Boots). 13. Petrolagar — 4 varieties. 14. Agarol. 15. Carbindon (Strong). 16. Bicolates. 17. Burroughs Wellcome Vegetable Laxative Pills. 18. Seidlitz Powder. 19. Eno's Fruit Salt. 20. Andrew's Fruit Salt. 21. Alembics Fruit Salt. 22. Frutal ko Saline. 23. Bishos's Salt. 24. Kruchon's Salt.

Senna Cascara, Pulvis Glycerize-co,
Seadlitz and Eno's Fruit Salt,
California Syrup of Figs,
Liquid paraffin and olive oil are mild laxatives.
They do not cause injury.
They can be safely given to pregnant women too.
Croton is the strongest purgative.
Aloes, Jalap, Scammony
Should never be given to pregnant women
And to patients who suffer from piles.
Senna should not be given
To nursing mothers,
Because babies will get diarrhoea.
Cultivate not enema habit, drug habit.
Take recourse to nature cure,
Fruits (figs, prunes, apples), vegetables,

Abdominal massage, hip-bath, mud plaster,
Exercise, Asanas, Suryanamaskar and Pranayamas.

Acrostic

Cascara is a mild laxative.
Olive oil softens the hard stools.
Nature-cure is highly beneficial.
Senna is a cheap purgative.
Tamarind acts as a laxative.
Irritant to purgatives are Jalap, Croton, Colocynth.
Phenolphthalein is suitable for children.
Aloes is a drastic purgative.
Tannin in Rhubarb causes after constipation.
Ipomoea or izabennsis is a cathartic.
Oleum Ricini produces after constipation.
Nature Mur is a Biochemical remedy for constipation.

How to Give an Enema

The enema is one of the oldest remedies for relieving constipation. Its use was known to the most ancient nations.

Enemas may be used for (1) evacuation of the bowels (enematic purgative), (2) to check diarrhoea or dysentry (constipating enema) and (3) to nourish the patient (nutrient enema). The fourth variety is saline enema. The fifth kind is medical enema.

More people need washing out than any other remedy. Avoid large quantities of water. The quantity of water should not exceed four pints. Two or three pints are quite sufficient. In some cases a pint is sufficient. This can be repeated.

For small quantities of water a glass syringe can be used. A douche-can is highly serviceable. Higginson's enema syringe is light, portable and suitable for travelling.

A No. 12 and No. 14 rubber catheter can be attached to the nozzle when a high enema is needed as in cases of long, continued constipation.

The tube attached to the can should be fitted with a rectal nozzle and all air in it should be let out before the nozzle is introduced into the rectum.

For purgative enema, plain, tepid water or soap water at the body temperature should be used.

Do not use too much force when you introduce the water inside the bowels. The water should be sent in slowly. If the water is introduced slowly, it will remain in the bowel for a long time and break up hard lumps of faeces.

Raise the can 2 or 3 feet above the level of bed.

After the water has been introduced a little time 5 or 10 minutes should be permitted to elapse before the water is expelled. This will insure more complete evacuation of the colon.

If the water is introduced too rapidly the colon resents and tries to expel it.

The flow of water should not be continuous but should be interrupted by pinching the tube the moment there is a slight feeling of distention or a desire for evacuation. After waiting a few seconds the sensation will fall off and more water may be allowed to enter. When the water is introduced slowly it has time to find its way upwards along the colon. In 5 or 10 minutes it will reach calcum. Movements occur in the bowel itself by which this ascent of the water is asserted. Reverse peristalsis begins in the transverse colon.

After introduction of water the tube should be taken out slowly. The anus should be kept plugged as long as is conveniently possible.

Let the patient remain on the left side. Raise the buttocks on a pillow. This helps the patient to retain the enema. Let him draw up his knees.

When you give enema avoid introducing air into the bowels. This can be done by allowing a small quantity of water to run out of the tube before inserting, so as to permit any air present there to escape.

He who uses enema should take bran, gar or other form of roughage with fresh fruits and green vegetables together with liquid paraffin or psyllium seed to supply the necessary bulk and lubrication.

Glycerine Enema:

For children a slight irritation near about the anus will expel lumps of hard stools. For this purpose a little glycerine may be introduced through the rectum. A special syringe with a bent ebonite nozzle is available for this purpose. A glass syringe will serve the purpose quite well.

Press the buttocks together with the left hand when you give an enema. Continue this for a short time after the removal of the nozzle.

Protect the bed by a Mackintosh or water-proof sheet.

Enema Glycerini:

Glycerine	4 fluid drachms
Water	1 fluid ounce
Mix.	

Enema Olei Olivae:

Olive oil	4 fluid ounces
Soft Soap	½ ounce
Water to	24 fluid ounces
Mix.	

Enema Saponis:

Soft Soap	1 ounce

Water to   24 fluid ounces
Mix.

Electro-Therapy

Electricity cooks food, cuts wood, drives motors, rolls papers, pumps water, gives light, moves fans and does so many things.

Electricity is used in the treatment of constipation, also.

Constipation which is due to irregular muscular action of the wall of the intestines may be treated by interrupted galvanic current.

A special electrode consisting of an India-rubber tube perforated by small holes, through which salt-water flows, is introduced into the intestines. The current is passed a few minutes every morning. Constipation is cured.

Have electric treatment under an expert only when all other natural remedies fail.

The galvanic current has a soothing and toning effect. It augments or increases metabolism. It stimulates and galvanises the functional activity of the parts through which it passes. The effect continues for days after application.

Psychic-Therapy

This body is a mould prepared by the mind
For its operation and all its activities.
Mind has great healing power.
It is a dynamo.
It is a mass of electricity.
A strong mind renovates and energises
The cells of the body and the intestines.
It stimulates the nerves and the
                              muscular coat of intestines.

Story of Purgatives

Purgatives are drugs that are prescribed to hasten evacuation of bowels by eliminating unnecessary or undesirable contents.

A laxative is a mild purgative. A purgative is stronger than a laxative. A drastic purgative is a very strong purgative, e.g., Jalap, colocynth. A hydragogue purgative is stronger than a drastic purgative, e.g., croton oil.

The above old classification into laxatives, purgatives, drastic purgatives and hydragogue purgatives is not satisfactory, because any of these drugs if given in sufficient amount may cause violent evacuation and tenesmus (griping pain). Division based upon the mode of action is more suitable.

Salines: Certain slowly diffusible salts, e.g., magnesium sulphate, sodium sulphate, and tartarate of sodium retain fluid in the bowel and thus increase the bulk of contents. Very watery motions are thus produced. The actions take place on the small and large intestines.

Colonic Purgatives: Rhubarb, Senna, Aloes and Cascara are called colonic purgatives. They take a fairly long time to act, about 10 to 12 hours They do not increase the peristalsis of the stomach or the small intestine, but only of the large intestine. They are certain in their action and produce a moderate amount of nearly painless purgation. They do not need bile for their action except rhubarb. Senna causes griping. Hence it should be given with carminatives like cinnamon or ginger.

Mild Purgatives: Confection of Senna and compound liquorice are mild purgatives.

Cascara Sagrada is bitter and is stomachic. It is a mild purgative. It is good for habitual constipation. It is best given at bed time to act in the following morning. A progressively increasing dose is not needed to be effective. There is very little griping. There is no after-constipation when it is stopped.

Cholagogue Purgatives: They definitely increase the secretion of bile and thus cause purgation, e.g., calomel, podophyllum (vegetable calomel).

Lubricants: Lubricants like liquid paraffin, olive oil act by softening the stools. They lubricate the intestinal canal. Passage of intestinal contents is facilitated. Mucilaginous vegetables like Isaphgul act in a similar manner. If given in excess they fail to produce the desired effect, because an unduly soft motion fails to stimulate peristalsis.

Irritant Purgatives: Irritant purgatives irritate the mucous membrane and consequently make it more sensitive to its contents. They increase the local reflex and thus accelerate peristalsis. They render the mucous membrane unduly sensitive to physiological Stimuli.

Castor oil, sulphur, jalap, colocynth, scammony, elaserium, gamboge, mercurials, anthracenes like rhubarb, senna, aloes, cascara sagrada, and drastic purgatives act in this way.

Castor oil acts upon the small bowel. The purgation comes after 3 or 4 hours.

Drastic purgatives like aloes, etc., exert uterine contractions. They should not be given to pregnant women.

Anthracena purgatives like aloes exert on the large intestines only. Defaecation takes place in half to one hour after their entrance into the caecum.

The interval between administration and purgation is 7 to 8 hours. That is the reason why it is usual to prescribe the anthrace purgatives for use at bed time.

Phenolphthalein acts slightly on the small bowel. It acts chiefly on the large intestine. Some is absorbed from the large intestine and reappears in the duodenum in the bile. It is soluble in the bile and alkaline contents of the intestine. Its effect is thus prolonged over 2 or 3 days in diminishing intensity.

The action of castor oil is rapid. It is usually given before breakfast in a dose of 1 or 2 ounces.

Colonel is given at night. The maximum dose is 5 grains. It must be washed out by a saline purgative in the morning, as it is important not to allow the mercury to be absorbed. It acts on the liver and throws out much bile in the small intestines.

Colocynth is mixed with hyoscyamus. Colocynth causes purgation and hyoscyamus which contains atropine paralyses the parasympathetic nerve endings and prevents excessive and painful contraction of the wall of the intestines.

Croton oil is given in a dose of one drop on a piece of sugar or mixed with butter as for example in uraemia convulsions when it is necessary to remove fluid from the body and the kidney is not able to do its function. Croton oil is the most powerful of all the purgatives.

Jalap, colocynth group acts on the small and large intestines. Purgation takes place in one to four hours.

Mercurial purgatives such as calomel, grey powder are valuable purgatives, as they are insoluble. The action of calomel is on both small and large intestines.

Some drugs such as pituitary extracts physostigmin and thyroid extract are neuro-muscular stimulants. They produce purgation by direct stimulation of the neuromuscular mechanism. They activate parasympathetic nerve endings, and increase intestinal movements. Posterior pituitary extract acts directly on the intestinal muscles. They are administered hypodermically. They are hypodermic purgatives. They are not really purgatives of general use. Thyroid extract given by the mouth corrects constipation by activating the metabolic process.

All powerful purgatives are followed by atony of the bowel and consequent constipation. This is highly marked after Rhubarb because of tannic acid content.

Rhubarb (Rhei) and senna render the urine deep yellow on account of the excretion of chrysophania acid. Phenolphthalein causes a pink colour if the urine is alkaline

Use of Purgatives: Purgatives relieve constipation. They ensure normal evacuation with ease.

They eliminate from the intestines the undesirable irritants or toxic substances.

They lower the blood-pressure.

They remove a collection of dropsical fluid. They remove the products of nitrogenous metabolism from the blood when the kidneys do not function properly.

Choice of Purgatives: The choice of purgatives for different patients is important. For babies and very small children, Liquor Magnesia Bicarbonate is or Fluid Magnesia is very good. For older children Cream of Magnesia or Mistura Magnesia Hydroxide is beneficial. Pure tasteless castor oil is also very useful for children.

If it is urgent to relieve constipation in a baby grey powder or Hydrargyrum cum creta is useful. Glycerine suppostrous are highly beneficial in combating against regular constipation of children.

Liquid paraffin, cascara are useful in chronic constipation of adults. Apples are very beneficial).

Senna and cascara stimulate the large bowel. Confection of Senna is useful.

Senna is a useful purgative for nursing mothers. This will not be secreted in the milk and produce purgation in the baby.

The colon is emptied well after a good purgative action. It takes 2 to 3 days to restore its normal tone.

Smoking

Smoking is not a remedy for constipation. It does not move the bowels. Smokers foolishly imagine that smoking causes free movement of the bowels. This is a terrible and sad mistake. Smoking poisons the system with nicotine. It causes irritable heart, tobacco amblyopia (a kind of eye disease) and countless diseases. Give up smoking at once and at one stroke and enjoy perfect health.

Chapter VI

PRESCRIPTIONS

1. Confections

Laxative Confections

1. Confection of Senna:

Powdered Senna	10
Powdered coriander	4
Figs	16
Tamarind pulp	12
Cassia pulp	12
Prunes	8
Extract of Liquorice	1½
Sugar	40
Water q.s. to	100

Dose: 60 to 120 grains. 1 to 2 teaspoonfuls.

2. Confection of Sulphur:

Precipitated sulphur	450
Acid Potassium tartrate	110
Tragacanth	5
Syrup	210
Tincture of orange	55
Glycerine	170

Dose: 60 to 120 grains

This is a good laxative useful in piles, haemorrohoids.

3.

Tamarind pulp	2 ounces
Prunes	2 ounces
Ext. Liquorice	2 drachms
Senna Leaves powder	1 ounce
Cardamom powder	½ ounce

Sugar	8 ounces

Make a confection. *Dose:* 1 teaspoonful.

4. An Effective Laxative:

Tamarind fruit	1 ounce
Dates	1 ounce
Milk	20 ounces

Boil and strain.

5. A Powerful Laxative:

Senna leaves powder	1 ounce
Prunes	1 ounce
Tamarind pulp	1 ounce
Cassia pulp	1 ounce
Cardamom powder	½ ounce
Sugar	6 ounces
Water	16 ounces

Dose: 1 tablespoonful.

2. Infusions

I

Infusion Senna *(Sonnamukki)*

Leaves of Cassia Lanceolata and Cassia Augustifolia. This is a good laxative. As there is no astringency they do not cause after-constipation.

Dose of senna leaves powder	4 drachms
Raisins	1 ounce
Ginger powder (Sonth)	1 drachm
Cloves powder	1 drachm
Boiling water	20 ounces

Allow to stand for 1 hour in a closed vessel and strain. *Dose:* 1 to 2 ounces. Add milk and sugar. It tastes like tea. It is easily taken by children. Avoid this in irritable condition of the bowels, piles and during pregnancy.

II
Infusion Senna

Senna powder   5
Cold water   half a tumbler.

Soak the powder in the cold water during the day. Strain and take it at bed time. Or soak it overnight. Strain and take it as the first thing in the early morning.

3. Mineral Waters

Carlsbad: This contains 13 grains of sulphate of soda to the tumbler with alkalis. *Dose:* 1 to 2 tumblers twice daily.

Friedrichshall: This contains 60 grains of magnesia and soda with alkalis. *Dose:* Half a tumblerful daily.

Hunyad Janos: This contains 200 grains of sulphates of soda and magnesia with alkalis. *Dose:* Quarter to half a tumbler. All of these are best given on an empty stomach.

Vichy: This is safe and helpful. This can be drunk freely. *Dose:* 2 to 4 ounces.

Pullna: *Dose:* 2 to 4 ounces.

4. Mixtures

1. White Mixture:

Magnesium carbonate   10 grains
Magnesium sulphate   1 drachm
Peppermint water to   1 ounce

A very useful saline aperient. Taken thrice daily, is used for some forms of dyspepsia and for constipation.

2. A Beneficial Mixture:

Tr. Nux vomica   m. 5
Tr. Belladonna   m. 5
Tr. Hyoscyanus   m. 10
Ext. Cas. Sagra Leg. add drachm 1
One Dose.

Belladonna and nux vomica in small dose undoubtedly promote peristalsis. Belladonna relaxes spasm.

3. **Black Draught: Mistura Sennae Co.:**
    Mag. Sulph.   25
    Liq. Extract of Liquorice   5
    Tr. card. co.   10
    Spt. ammonia aromaticus   5
    Fresh infusion of senna to make 100
    Dose: 1 to 2 fluid ounces. This is a good purgative.

4. **Mistura Acidi Sulphuric cum Opio:**
    Dilute Sulphuric Acid   10 m.
    Tincture of Opium   10 m.
    Cinnamon Water to   1 fluid ounce.
    Mix. *Dose:* 1 Fluid ounce.

5. Pills
Laxative and Purgative Pills

1. **Calomel, Colocynth and Hyoscyamus Pill:**
    Calomel   1½ grs.
    Extract of hyoscyamus   1 grn.
    Compound Extract of colocynth   2½ grs.
    A good purgative pill: one or two at night.

2. **Nux Vomica and Belladonna Pill:**
    Alcoholic extract of belladonna ¼ grn.
    Extract of nux vomica   ¼ grn.
    Extract of aloes   1 grn.
    Used in constipation due to lack of muscular power in the bowel. One or two at night.

3. **Rhubarb and Mercury Pill:**
    Mercury pill   2½ grs.
    Compound rhubarb pill   2½ grs.
    A good purgative pill: is very kind. One or two at night.

4. **Pilula Colocynthidis et Hydrargyri:**

Compound Pill of Colocynth   1½ grs.
Pill of Mercury   1 grn.
Extract of Hyoscyamus   ½ grn.
Mix for 1 pill. *Dose:* 1 or 2 pills.

5. **Pilula Cascara Sagrada Col:**
Dry Extract of Cascara Sagrada 2½ grs.
Powdered Capsicum   ¼ grn.
Dry Extract of Nux Vomica   ¼ grn.
Dry Extract of Bellabonna   ¼ grn.
Rectified Spirit (90 per cent) Sufficient quantity
Mix for 1 pill.

6. **Pill Aloin Co:**
Aloin   ¼ grn.
Strychnim   1/60 grn.
Ext. Belladonna   1/16 grn.
Ext. Cascara   ½ grn.
One Pill, thrice daily.

7. **A Vegetable Pill:**
Pill. Colocynth Co   1 gr.
Pill. Rhei Co.   1 gr.
Ext. Hyoscyamus   ½ gr

Make one pill. *Dose:* 2 at bed-time. A very useful vegetable pill.

8. **Aloes and Nux Vomica Pill:**
Aloes   2 grs.
Dry Ext. of Nux Vomica   ¼ gr.
Dry Ext. of Belladonna   1/6 gr.
Dose: 1 pill.

9. **Pilula Aloes et Ferri (Pill of aloes and Iron):**
Exsiccated Ferrous Sulphate
Aloes
Cinnamon

Cardamom
Ginger

Dose: 4 to 8 grains. Useful when there is anaemia or poverty of blood. Aloes must not be given when pregnancy, piles or excessive menstruation exist.

10. **Pilula Aloes** *(Aloes Pill):*
    Aloes
    Hard Soap
    Oil of Caraway
    Syrup of Glucose
    Dose: 4 to 8 grains

11. **Colocynth and Hyoscyamus Pill:**

Colocynth	12.5 grs.
Aloes	25 grs.
Scammony resin	25 grs.
Dry Extract of Hyoscyamus	12.5 grs.

Dose: 4 to 8 grains. Excellent purgative. This should not be given in pregnancy and on irritable condition of stomach and intestines.

12. **Cathartic Pill:**

Calomel	3 grs.
Ext. Hyoscyamus	2 grs.
Ext. Colocynth Co.	5 grs.

Mix and divide into two pills for one dose.

13. **Cathartic Compound Pills** (Parke Davis & Co.)

Ext. Colocynth Co.	1½ grs.
Calomel	1 gr.
Resin of Jalap	⅓ gr.
Powder Gamboge	¼ gr.

An excellent purgative pill.   *Dose:* 1 to 3.

14. **Cathartic Vegetable:** (Parke Davis & Co.)

Ext. Colocynth Co.	1 gr.

Ext. Hyoscyamus   ½ gr.
Resin of Jalap   ⅓ gr.
Ext. Leptandra   ¼ gr.
Podophyllun Resin   ¼ gr.
Oil of peppermint   ⅛ gr.
A milk purgative pill.   *Dose:* 1 to 2.

6. Powders
Laxative Powders

1. Myrobalans (Harad)   1 drachm
   Fennel fruit (Bari Sonp) 2 drachm
   Sugar   2 drachm
   This is a good laxative powder.

2. **Kaladana Powder:**
   Black seed (Kaladana) in fine powder 1 drachm
   Powdered ginger   10 grains
   One dose. This is a good purgative.

3. **Pulvis Jalapae Co.**
   Pulvis Jalap   5 ozs.
   Acid Pot. Tart.   9 ozs.
   Ginger   1 oz.
   Mix well. *Dose:* 20 to 60 grains. A good purgative.

4. Powder of Senna leaves   10 grains
   Liquorice (Mulathi)   10 grains
   Sulphur (purified)   5 grains
   Cardamom   5 grains
   Dose: 1 powder. This is one of the best laxative powders.

5. **Pulvis Glycyrrhiza Co.**
   Senna.   16 grs.
   Liquorice root   16 grs.
   Fennel   8 grs.
   Sublimed sulphur 8 grs.
   Sugar   58 grs.

Dose: 6 – 120 grains. This is a safe laxative powder. Take this at bed-time. It is very useful in Piles or Haemorrhoids.

6. **Pulvis Effervescens Compositus** – Dose 1925. grs. Seidlitz powder. Take Soda tartrate 7.5 grms. (115.5 grs.) Sodii Bicarb. 2.5 grms. (38.5 grs.), mix these two and wrap in a blue paper; Tartaric acid 2.5 grms. (38.5 grs.) wrap in a white paper. Dissolve the powder in blue paper in 8 oz. of water and add the powder in white paper and drink while effervescing.

7. Salt
Sodii Et Potassii Tartras (Na KC$_4$ H$_4$O$_6$, 4H$_2$O)

Syn. Soda Tartrate, Rochelle Salt.

Prepared by neutralising potash tartrate with sodium bicarbonate. It occurs in colourless crystals soluble 1 in 1½ of water.

Dose: – 120 to 240 grs. – 8-16 grms.

Laxatives and Purgatives: Hygienic measures must be observed, and bad habits of life corrected. Diet is an essential factor, especially insufficiency of bulky food. Gentle massage; high-frequency current. The drug must be selected with reference to the etiology or cause.

Treat different varieties of impaired digestion; starch, with Taka-Diastase; protein with Lactated Pepsin, Panteric C.C.T., Panteric Compound.

Remedies to unload the bowel: – Purgative salts, Cathartic Comp., Amerol.

Drugs to influence intestine to normal activity – Cascara Sagrada F.E., Cascara Evacuant, Phenolphthalein Comp. S.C.T, Alophen Pill cholelith Pill.

Measures to clear the colon – Enemata and Glycerine Suppositorics.

To establish and maintain peristalsis, Cascara Sagrada is

unrivalled, particularly in the form of the fluid extract Cascara Sagrada Aromatic, Amerol, or Milk of Magnesia.

Cathartic Vegetable Pill is gentle and effective. Pitressin.

Aperients

Intestinal Lubricant: Amerol.

Mild or Laxative: Cascara Aromatic, Cascara Evacuant, Cathartic Comp. Pill, Milk of Magnesia, Rhubarb Comp. Tincture.

Cathartics: Aloes, Alophen Pill, Cascara, Euonymin, Jalap, Phenolphthalein, Podophyllin, Panteric Comp.

Hydragogues: Colocynth, Jalap, Sodium Sulphate, Magnesium Sulphate.

Milk of Magnesia: A preparation of milk-like appearance and consistency containing about 32 grains of magnesium hydrate in each fluid ounce.

Milk of Magnesia possesses several advantages over magnesium carbonate, also over calcined and fluid magnesia, both in therapeutic efficiency and in convenience of administration. An efficient antacid and laxative suitable for children as well as adults.

Dose as an antacid, etc., from ½ to 1 fluid drachm (2 to 4 c.c.) as a laxative, from 1 to 4 fluid drachms (4 to 15 c.c.) in water.

Molevac: (a mechanico-physiological tonic-laxative).

A combination of Liquid Petrolatum of high viscosity with Malt Extract and Cascara Evacuant, P.D. & Co. (12 minims in each fluid ounce).

Molevac is a combined peristaltic stimulant and intestinal lubricant which is particularly useful in those cases of chronic constipation in which the merely mechanical effect of liquid petrolatum proves insufficient and needs to be supplemented by the administration of a physiological laxative.

Dose — From one teaspoonful, upwards, as found necessary.

Chapter VII

PURGATIVES

(Virechani)

The following is a list of purgative drugs: Myrobalan, Thandrikkai, Nellimulli, Croton only in very small doses; Bastard Teak (seeds of Butea Frondosa), Jalap (purified chivatai roots,) Vaivilangam, Brahmi leaves, Induppu (Rock salt), Mudakothan leaves, Senna, Kadugurohini and Chathurakkalli.

The genuine drug *Cascara Sagrada* stored under the proper conditions has proved one of the greatest additions to the armamentarium of the physician. It is a remedy of very high repute in the treatment of chronic constipation. The great advantage of Cascara lies in the fact that it causes soft and painless evacuations of the bowels and after its discontinuance there is no tendency to constipation. Even in the worst cases, there is no necessity at all to increase the dose. After a time the drug can be entirely discontinued.

Liquid Extract of Cascara Sagrada   drachm ½
Water   oz 1

Mix: To be taken at bed-time. The dose of the cascara may be gradually increased to 1 drachm

The use of purgatives, when continued for any length of time, tends to cause constipation. In time, the bowels become so used to this artificial stimulus that they are unable to act without it.

A cup of tea in the early morning acts as a laxative and moves the bowels freely. A small quantity of *mel* i.e., honey taken just before retiring to bed proves beneficial. Chronic constipation arises also from the in judicious administration of purgatives. Pills containing mercury should be avoided as they eat away the gums and cause early loss of teeth. The application of electricity is made use of in the treatment of chronic constipation. The movements of the bowels are due to the alternate contractions and dilatations of their muscular coats. This peculiar sort of wave-like movement of the bowels is termed *peristaltic* or *vermicular* movement. In constipation this movement is paralysed and the faecal matter accumulates. A current of electricity passed through the bowels removes the temporary paralysis of the peristaltic movement and effects free movement of the bowels. A confection made out of the pulp of bael fruit *(aegle marmelos* also, *stone apple)* by mixing with a small quantity of honey is of great service. Figs, fruits, dates all exercise a soothening influence in the bowels and cause free movement. The infusion of *chirata* stimulates the liver, causes free secretion of the bile and is a remedy of high value in chronic constipation. Persons suffering from long standing constipation may take with much advantage one or two drachms of compound liquarice powder at bed-time.

Purgative *mineral* waters as *Hunyadi Janos,* Friedrichshall, *carlshad,* Pullna, etc., are of great service. They must be taken before breakfast. An enema of castor oil, glycerine, or soap and water immediately brings about evacuation of the bowels.

Let us turn out attention to the Aryan store of drugs. We can find there Confection of Myrobalan, Gammara Confection, Jalap Confection, Tesavara lehyam, Sukhabhedi Confection, Sukhabhedi salt, Sukhabhedi oil, Myrobalan Ghee, Haibathi Choorna, Vibhakti Choorna,

Nilavahai Choorna, Vibhodhi Lehyam, Narthangai, Lehyam, Mudakathan Lehyam, *sherbet* obtained from fresh red rose petals, are remedies of high value in the treatment of constipation.

I

Drugs that produce copious watery evacuation from the bowels: — Common Milk Hedge (Euphorbia Nivulia), Ilaikkalli (Tamil), Snuhipatram (Sanskrit), Thohar (Hindi). The leaf, milk and root are purgatives.

Milk Hedge plant (Euphorbia Tirucalli) — Snuhi (Sanskrit), Barki-thohar (Hindi).

Yellow champa (Michelia Champaea) — Shanbagam (Tamil), Champaka (Sanskrit), Champa (Hindi). The root is a purgative.

Jequirety (Abrus precatorius) — Gunja (Sanskrit), Gunj (Hindi).

Bengal hemp (Crotalaria Juncea) — Chanappu (Tamil), Pulivanji (Sanskrit), San (Hindi). The leaf is a purgative.

Indian Ladurnam (Cassia fistula) — Sarakhonrai (Tamil), Aragvadham (Sanskrit), Amaltas (Hindi). The seed, root-bark, fruit-pulp are purgatives.

Ficus Nolycarpa — Chiru peyatti (Tamil).

Custard apple (Anona Squamosa) — Seetha (Tamil), Subha (Sanskrit), Sharifah (Hindi). The root is a purgative.

Chukkankai (Tamil), Thummattikai (Tamil). The leaf and root are purgatives.

Bottle gourd (Lagenaria Vulgaris) — Churai (Tamil), Alabu (Sanskrit), Lauki (Hindi). The leaf is a purgative.

Tigers milk tree (Execaria Agallocha) — Tillai (Tamil), Ugaru (Sanskrit), Gangiya (Hindi).

Alhagi Maurorum, Thurinjibin (Tamil).

Nilavamanakku (Tamil), Lal-cheranda (Hindi).

Country Senna or Indian or Tinnevelly Senna (Cassia lanceolata) – Nilavarai (Tamil), Sunnamakhi (Hindi).

Croton (Croton Tiglium) – Nervalan (Tamil), Danthi (Sanskrit), Jamalgotta (Hindi)

Ribbed lutfa (Cucumis accutangula) – Pirkku (Tamil), Kosavathee (Sanskrit), Turai (Hindi). The seed is a purgative.

Brown Indian Hemp (Hibiscus Cannabinus) – Pulich-chirukirai (Tamil), Machika Phalamla (Sanskrit), Patsan (Hindi). The leaf is a purgative.

Toothbrush tree (Palvadora Indica) – Perungkalarva (Tamil), Barapilu (Hindi). The fruit is a purgative.

Negro Coffee (Cassia Occidentalis) – Peyavarai (Tamil), Kasamarda (Sanskrit), Kasunda (Hindi).

Sansevieria Roxburghiana – Marul (Tamil), Moorva (Sanskrit), Murhari (Hindi).

Ringworm shrub (Cassia Alata) – Vandukulli (Tamil), Dadrughna (Sanskrit), Dadmurdan (Hindi).

Cleomepruticosa – Vizhudi (Tamil).

Bitter gourd (Cucumis Trigonus) – Kattuthumatti (Tamil), Vishala (Sanskrit), Jangli Indarayan (Hindi). The root is a purgative.

Trichosanthe Cucumerina – Kattupeipudal (Tamil), Patola (Sanskrit), Jangli-chichonda (Hindi). The root is a purgative.

Mesuua Ferrea – Chirunagappu (Tamil), Naga-kesara (Sanskrit), Naga-Kesar (Hindi). The unripe fruit is a purgative.

II

• Aloes • Alu Bokara – Prunes • Arachis oil • Bael
• Bringaraj – Karasalanganni (Tamil) • Castor oil
• Gamboge – Resin of Carcinia pictoria • Har or Chhoti

Har—Chubelic myrobalans ● Indian Aloes (Kartazhai) (Tamil), Kumari (Sanskrit), Ghikauvar (Hindi) ● Isafgul ● Kaladana—Seeds of Impomoea hedercea ● Leaves of pine apple ● Myrobalan ● Nux Vomica ● Oleander— Alari (Tamil), Karaveera (Sanskrit) ● Rhubarb—Rheus emoli roots ● Sendha Nimak—Rock Salt ● Senna— Leaves of Cassia lanceolata and Cassia angustifolia ● Sulphur—Gandhak ● Superb-Lily—Kalappai Kizhanghu (Tamil), Sukrapushpika (Sanskrit) ● Tamarind —Imli—Pulp of fruit ● Turpeth Root—Pithori, Root of Impomoea turpethum ● Worm-killer—Adutindapalai (Tamil), Maspurisha (Sanskrit).

Har – Chubelle myrobalans. • Indian Aloe (Karnazian)
(Tamil), Kumari (Sanskrit), Ghikanvar (Hindi) • Isabgul
– Kaladana – Seed of Impomoea hederacea • Leaves of
pine apple • Myrobalans – Haritaki – Homica • Oleander –
Alari (Tamil), Karavira (Sanskrit), • Rhubarb - Rheus
emoli roots – Sendha Namak—Rock Salt • Sonea –
Leaves of Cassia lanceolata and Cassia angustifolia
• Sulphur – Gandhak • Superb Lily – Kalappai
Kizhanghu (Tamil), Kalihari (Sanskrit) • Tamarind
Impomoca turpethum • Worm-killer

Chapter VIII

AYURVEDIC MEDICINES

Laxatives

(Laghuvirechani)

Laxatives are medicines that loosen the bowel. They are mild purgatives.

Agati grandiflora – Agathi (Tamil), Agastya (Sanskrit), Agti (Urdu). The leaf is a laxative.

Walnut Seed (Juglans Regia) – Akrothuvitai (Tamil), Akshodas (Sanskrit), Akrot (Hindi). The seed is a mild laxative.

Glycerrihizae Radix (Abrus Precatorius) – Ati-maduram (Tamil), Yashti Madhukam (Sanskrit), Mulathi (Hindi).

Country fig (Ficus Racemosa) – Atti (Tamil), Udumbara (Sanskrit), Gular (Urdu). The fruit is a laxative.

The Wester-lettuce (Tropical Duckweed or Pistia Stratiotes) – Antaratamarai or Akasathamarai (Tamil), Kumbhika, Variparni (Sanskrit), Jal-kumbhi (Hindi). The leaf is a laxative.

Four O'clock flower (Mirabilis Jalapa) – Andimalli (Tamil), Sandhya-raga (Sanskrit), Gule-aabbas (Hindi). The root is a laxative.

Australian asthma weed (Euphorbia Pilulifera) – Ammanpacharisi (Tamil), Kshiriniraga (Sanskrit), Dudhi (Hindi).

The Peepul tree, the sacred fig (Ficus Religiosa) – Arasu (Tamil), Aswatha (Sanskrit), Pipal (Hindi). The seed is a laxative.

Country goose berry (Avverrhoea acida) – Arunelli (Tamil), Chelmeri (Hindi). The seed is a laxative.

Sageleaved Alangium (Alangium Decaptalum) – Azhinjil (Tamil), Amkolam (Sanskrit), Akola (Hindi).

Unripe Pineapple (Ananas Sativvus) – Anasikay (Tamil), Ananas (Hindi).

Castor oil – Amanakkuennai (Tamil), Yeranda-Tailam (Sanskrit), Arandikatel (Hindi). The oil is a laxative.

The seed of the Banyan tree (Ficus Bengalensis) – Alamaram (Tamil), Vata (Sanskrit), Bargad (Hindi). The seed is a laxative.

Purumus communis var Institia – Alpogadapazham (Tamil), Alu-bokhara (Hindi).

Linseed (Lepidium Sativum) – Ali-verai (Tamil), Chandrasura (Sanskrit), Chansar (Hindi). The seed is a laxative.

Almond sweet (Amygdala dulus) – Vadumari (Tamil), Badarna (Sanskrit), Badam (Hindi).

Potato (Solanum Tuberosum) – Urulaikkizhangu (Tamil), Alu (Hindi).

Cassia Tora – Usiththakarai (Tamil), Chakramarda (Sanskrit), Chakunda (Hindi).

Mudar (Calotropis gigantea) – Erukku (Tamil), Arka (Sanskrit). The leaf is a laxative.

Prenanthes Sarmentosa – Ezhuttanippundu (Tamil).

Sesamum Indicum (Gingely oil-plant) – Ellu (Tamil), Tilam (Sanskrit), Til (Hindi). The seed is a laxative.

Briyonia Laciniosa, Iyvirali.

Bengalgram (Chicken pea), (Cicer Arientum) – Kadalai (Tamil), Chanaka (Sanskrit), Chana (Hindi). The juice of the leaf is a laxative.

Cocculus Villosus—Kattukodi (Tamil), Vasanavalli (Sanskrit), Jamtika-patta (Hindi).

Sugarcane (Saecharum officinarum)—Karumbu (Tamil), Ikshu (Sanskrit), Ganna (Hindi). The sugarcane juice is a laxative.

Mixed greens—Kalavaikkeerai (Tamil).

Indian coral tree (Erythrina Indica)—Kaliyana Murukku (Tamil), Parijataka (Sanskrit), Mandar (Hindi). The leaf is a laxative.

Kattuch-chatakuppai (Tamil).

Babchi seeds (Psoralia Corylifolia)—Karpokarisi (Tamil), Vakuchi (Sanskrit), Bavanchiyan (Hindi).

The Mangoose plant (Ophiorhiza Munghos)— Keeripundu (Tamil), Nagasugandha (Sanskrit), Sarahati (Hindi).

Amaranthus Gangeticus—Keerai-thandu (Tamil), Harithaka (Sanskrit).

The Mexican poppy, the yellow thistle (Argemone Mexicana)—Brahmadandi (Sanskrit), Bharbhand (Hindi). The seed is a laxative.

Jequirity (Abrus precatorius)—Kuntri (Tamil), Gunja (Sanskrit), Gunj (Hindi). The leaf is a laxative.

Sago palm (Caryota palm)—Kuntharpanai (Tamil), Mari (Hindi).

Amygdula (amara)—Bitter almond, Kaippu Vadumai (Tamil).

Baasella Alba (White basil or Indian spinach)— Koddippasalaik keerai (Tamil), Potaki (Sanskrit), Myalkibhaji (Hindi).

Cassiafistula (Indian Ladurnam),—Pudding-pipe tree, Sarakonrai (Tamil), Aragvadham (Sanskrit), Amaltas (Hindi). The leaf and bark are laxatives.

Trianthema decandra — Sattichcharanai (Tamil); Punarnava (Sanskrit).

Chamomile flowers (Chrysanthemum Indicum) — Samantippu (Tamil), Shevmntika-pushpam (Sanskrit), Gulchinika-phul (Hindi).

Acacia Concinna — Cheeyak kai (Tamil), Saptala (Sanskrit), Kochi (Hindi).

Ficus Carica (Fig) — Shimai-Atti (Tamil), Angurah (Sanskrit), Anjir (Urdu). The fruit is a laxative.

Shoe flower (Hibiscus Rosa) — Sinensis, Japa (Sanskrit), Jasun (Hindi).

Cocco (Arum Colocasia) — Cheppankizhanghee (Tamil), Kachu (Hindi).

Maize (Holcus Sorghum) — Cholam (Tamil).

Cape gooseberry (Physalis Meninia) — Thakkali (Tamil), Tankari (Sanskrit), Tulalipati (Hindi).

Chinese gooseberry (Averrhoa Carmbola) — Ramaraththam (Tamil), Karmaranga (Sanskrit), Karmaranga (Hindi).

Common fumitory (Fumaria parviflora) — Thara (Tamil), Parpat (Sanskrit), Kshetra Parputi (Hindi).

Beleric Myrobalans (Terminalia Belerica) — Thantri (Tamil), Vebheethaki (Sanskrit), Bhairah (Hindi).

Grapes (Vitis Vinifera) — Thrakshi (Tamil), Draksha (Sanskrit), Munakha (Hindi). The fruit is a laxative.

The country mallow (Abutilon Indicum) — Thuththi (Tamil), Kankatika (Sanskrit), Kanghi (Hindi).

Leucus Aspera — Thumbai (Tamil), Dronapushpi (Sanskrit), Guma Madhupati (Hindi).

Cocoanut palm (Cocos Nucifera) — Thenku-maram (Tamil), Narikela (Sanskrit), Nariyal (Hindi). The tender cocoanut juice and the juice of the pulp are laxatives.

Ipomea digitata—Nilappusini (Tamil), Vidrai (Sanskrit), Bilai-khand (Hindi).

Thyme-leaves Gratiola (Herpestis Monniera)—Nirbrahmi (Tamil), Mandukaparni (Sanskrit), Barambhi (Hindi)

Indian gooseberry (Phyllanthus Emblica)—Nelli (Tamil), Amalaki (Sanskrit), Amlika (Hindi). The fruit is a laxative.

Celosia Albida—Pannaikkeerai (Tamil), Pila-murghka (Hindi).

Papaw tree (Carica Papaya)—Pappai (Tamil), Papeeta (Hindi). The fruit is a laxative.

Indian Cotton plant (Gossypium Indicum)—Parutti (Tamil), Carpasa (Sanskrit), Kapas (Hindi). The seed is a laxative.

Jack tree (Artocarpus Integrifolia)—Pala (Tamil), Pansa (Sanskrit), Kathal (Hindi). The fruit is a laxative.

Bastard Teak (Butea Frondosa)—Palasu (Tamil), Palash (Sanskrit), Dhara (Hindi). The seed is a laxative.

Night Jasmin (Nyctanthes Arbor-tristis)—Pavalamalli or Parijatam (Tamil), Parijataka (Sanskrit), Harsinghar (Hindi). The leaf is a laxative.

Justicia Madurensis—Parattaikeerai (Tamil).

Mollugo Cerviana—Parpatakam (Tamil), Parpatakam (Sanskrit), Paph-Jhad (Hindi).

Bitter Gourd (Momordica charantia)—Pakal (Tamil), Karavalli (Sanskrit), Karela (Hindi). The fruit is a laxative.

Pavetta Indica—Pavattai (Tamil), Pappanna (Sanskrit), Kankra (Hindi).

Ruellia Secunda—Parchorikkeerai (Tamil).

Melochia Corchorifolia—Pinnakkukeerai (Tamil).

Thyme-leaved gratiola (Gratiola Monieri) – Piramiya – Vazhukhai (Tamil).

Gold Thread (Thalictrum Foliolosum) – Pitharohini (Tamil), Peetharohinee (Sanrkrit), Pilijari (Hindi). The root is a laxative.

Poon tree (Sterculia Foetida) – Pinarimaram (Tamil), Poothaekam (Sanskrit), Jungli Badam (Hindi).

Tamarind tree (Tamarindus Indica) – Puli (Tamil), Tintrini (Sanskrit), Imli (Hindi). The fruit is a laxative.

Polygala telephioides – Peria-Nankai (Tamil).

Tooth-brush tree (Palvadora Indica) – Perung-kalarva (Tamil). The flower is a laxative. The fruit is a purgative.

Asafoetida (Ferula Asafoetida) – Perungkayam (Tamil), Hingu (Sanskrit), Hing (Hindi).

Gisekia Pharnaceoidas – Manalikkirai (Tamil), Valuka (Sanskrit), Balukasag (Hindi).

Bauhinia Perpurea – Mantharai (Sivappu, red) (Tamil), Kanchanara (Sanskrit), Kachnar (Hindi). The flower and root are laxatives.

Manna (Tamrix callica) – Manna (Tamil), Jhavuka (Sanskrit), Jhan (Hindi). This milk is a laxative.

Mango tree (Mangifera Indica) – Amra Vriksha (Sanskrit), Amkaped (Hindi). The unripe fruit and the fruit are laxatives.

Three leaved caper (crataeva religeosa) – Mavilangu (Tamil), Pashugandha (Sanskrit), Tapia (Hindi). The bark of the tree and the bark of the root are laxatixes.

Ipomoea Candicans – Musuttai (Tamil).

Winter cherry or heart pea, balloon-vine (cardiospermum halicacabum) – Mudakkatran (Tamil), Karnasphota (Sanskrit), Kanphata (Hindi).

Garden Radish (Raphanus Sativus) — Mullangi (Tamil), Moolaka (Sanskrit), Muli (Hindi).

The red silk-cotton tree (Bombax Malabaricum or Bombax Hepataphylla) — Mulilavu (Tamil), Kantaka-Shalmali (Sanskrit), Ragai-semal (Hindi). The flower is a laxative.

Boerhaavia diffusa — Mukkiratti (Tamil), Punarnava (Sanskrit), Gadha-purna (Hindi).

Sesuvium Adscendens — Vankaravallai keerai (Tamil).

The plantain tree (Musa Sapientum) — Vazhai (Tamil), Kadali (Sanskrit). The fruit is a laxative.

Bael tree (Aegle Marmelos) — Vilvam (Tamil), Bilva (Sanskrit), Bel (Hindi). The fruit is a laxative.

Fenugreek (Trigonella Foenum) — Vendayam (Tamil), Methi (Sanskrit), Methi (Hindi). The leaf is a laxative.

Adenema Hissopifolia — Vellarugu (Tamil).

The Indian Kino tree (Ptero-carpus) (Marsupium) — Vengai (Tamil), Asanam (Sanskrit), Bijasar (Hindi). The gum is a laxative.

Groundnut or peanut — Verkadalai or Nilakadalai (Tamil), Buchanaka (Sanskrit), Mungphali (Hindi).

Chapter IX
CATHARTIC

(Virechanakari)
Strong Purgatives

Rhubarb – Iraval Chinni (Tamil), Reval-chinni (Sanskrit), Revand Chini (Hindi).

Plumeria, Alba – Ezhattalari (Tamil), Kshira-champaka (Sanskrit), Gulchin (Hindi). The root and its bark are cathartics.

Hicrorrhiza Kurroa – Katukurohani (Tamil), Katurohani (Sanskrit). The root is a cathartic.

Monkey pax tree – Mallotus Phillippiensis) – Kamela (Tamil), Kampilla (Sanskrit), Kamala (Hindi).

Aloe Indica – Rattabolam (Tamil), Kariabolam (Tamil), Shottu-katrazhai (Tamil), Rakthabolam (Sanskrit), Musambar (Hindi).

Horse gram, black (Cassia Absus) – Kattukollu (Tamil), Vana-kulutha (Sanskrit), Chaksu (Hindi).

Indian acalypha, Cat's struggle (Acalypha Indica) – Kuppai-meni (Tamil), Arithamanjarie (Sanskrit), Kuppi (Hindi). The root is a cathartic.

Trichosanthes Palmata – Kurattai (Tamil), Mahakala (Sahskrit), Lal-indrayan (Hindi). The root is a cathartic.

Kaladana seeds (Ipomoea Hederaceae) – Kodikkak-kattan vitai (Tamil), Kaladanah (Hindi).

Oil from the fruit of Bengal Walnut (Aleuritis Triloba) – Nattu Akrottu oil (Tamil), Akrota (Sanskrit), Akrot (Hindi).

Indian Mulberry (Morissda citrifolia) — Nuna (Tamil), Achuka (Sanskrit), Acchi (Hindi). The root is a cathartic.

The leaves and bark of Common bead tree, the Persian Lilac, Mali-Vembu (Tamil), Maha-nimba or Parvatha Nimba (Sanskrit), Bakayan (Hindi).

Ayurvedic Purgatives

Anaha

Purgatives, e.g., Shiva-kshar-pachan
Choorna and tablets   5 grains
Abhayadi Modak tikdi
Swadhista Virechana Choorna or tikdi
Siva-kshar Pachan Vati   5 grains
4 to 12 tablets with water twice a day.

Abhyadi Modak 5 grains. Dose: one tablet to be taken with warm water. Each tablet contains ½ grain chota seeds. Chief ingredients are Trivrit, sugar, Danti seeds, Pippali, Amalak, etc. Not to be given to pregnant women, old and weak persons and young children.

Swadhista Virechana Choorna: Dose: 60 to 120 grains to be taken at bed time. Chief ingredients are Yastimadhu, Shatapushpi, Markandi, Gandhaka and sugar.

Useful in piles, constipation, prolapsus anus, fissure of anus.

Swadhista V. tablet: 15 grains. Dose: 2 to 8 tablets with water at bed-time.

Shiva-kshar Pachan Choorna: Dose ½ to 1 tola to be taken twice a day with water. Chief ingredients are Shiva, Soda-bi-carb and Hingu-astak. Useful in constipation, indigestion and other bowel complaints.

Ayurvedic Prescriptions for Constipation
1. Panchasakaar Choorna

Re: Sonf Powder   1 Tola
    Suddha Suhaga Powder   1 Tola
    Saindhawa Namak (Salt) Powder   1 Tola
    Sanayapatti Powder   2 Tolas
    Shiva (Haritaki) Powder   2 Tolas

(Suhaga can be purified by keeping it in an iron pan over the fire).

Take Khichidi at night before taking this medicine. Take 1 Tola of this powder and with a little water (warm). Also take hot water in the morning.

2. Draakashaadi Leha

Re: Chotee Pippali   1 Tola
    Nisotha   4 Tolas
    Hararh   1 Tola

Make these three into a fine powder. Take 5 Tolas of raisins. Make them into paste. Add these two in 8 tolas of good honey. Mix them nicely. Keep this Lehyam in a bottle. 2 Tolas of this Lehyam can be taken with 2 seers of hot milk, every day.

3. Triphala Choorna

Re: Hararh Powder   2 Tolas
    Baherha Powder   1 Tola
    Awala Powder   1 Tola
    Saindhawa Namak (Salt) Powder   2 Tolas

Strain the powder. Take Khichidi at night. One tola of this powder may be taken before going to bed at night in a little hot water. After half-an hour of taking this powder, another glass of hot water can be taken.

4. Draakshaadi Kwath
Re: Boil 5 Tolas of Munakka (big raisins) in 40 Tolas of

water, till it is reduced to 20 Tolas. Filter the water and add the Nisotha Powder to that. Drink it before going to bed.

5. Triphalaadi Ghrita

Re: Boil 4 Tolas of Hararh, 2 tolas of Baherha and 2 Tolas of Awala in 64 Tolas of water. Reduce it to one-fourth. Filter. Add 5 Tolas of Ghee to it and boil it in mild fire, till the water is evaporated. Keep it in a bottle. 2 Tolas of this Ghee may be taken with 2 tola of Sugar.

6. Pippalyaadi Leha

Re: Nisotha   1 Tola
    Indra Jaun   1 Tola
    Pippali   2 Tolas
    Sonth   2 Tolas
    Munakka   1 Tola

Boil down to one half. Filter and make it cool. Add honey to equal proportion add mix with 8 tolas of Trikatu Choorna. Dose: 2 Tolas.

7. Abhayaadi Modak

Re: i.   Hararh, Black pepper, Sonth, Vayaviding, Awala, Pippala, Pipalamoola, Daalcheeni, Tejpaat and Nagar Motha (one part each);
    ii. Root of Danti (two parts);
    iii. Nisotha (eight parts);
    iv. Sugar (6 parts);

Powder these and strain. Add honey to equal proportion. Prepare balls (Laddus) of one tola each. Dose: one ball every morning with cold water.

8. Soonthyadi Choorna

Re: Saindhawa Namak (Salt) Powder   1 Tola
    Sonth Powder   1 Tola
    Nisotha Powder   1 Tola

Strain. Add 2½ Tolas of lemon juice and stir nicely. Keep

it in a bottle. Dose: 1 Tola of powder every day with hot water.

9. Triphalaadi kwaath

Re: Boil down 5 tolas of Triphala Choorna in 20 Tolas of water to one-half. Filter it. Add 2 tolas Triketu Choorna (Sonth, Mircha, Pippal) to it. Dose: Drink it before going to the bed.

Chapter X

NATUROPATHIC TREATMENT OF CONSTIPATION

Introduction: Conditions which help constipation are too numerous in this machine age. This machine age instead of giving relief to the man, has created many diseases. The fault does not lie with machine, but with man; because instead of becoming the master of the machine, he has become a slave to it. Excess of anything is bad, so also excessive use of machinery has brought upon man many evils.

Unnatural Living is at the root of loss of health and vitality. Instead of living in pure air, a man has to live, work in a congested area, has to work more for gaining sufficient money to maintain himself and his family. Ordinary man cannot get sufficient leisure. He is required to work at odd times when he is not expected to work. He has to take meals at a time when he is not hungry. He has to wake up late at night owing to overwork or arrears of work. In short he has to work against Nature and so has to suffer consequences in the form of loss of health and vitality.

These causes are beyond the control of man. He cannot change the drift of the existing circumstances. He must change and adapt himself, otherwise there is no other go.

The cumulative effect of wrong living brings on constipation very slowly so much so that it is not felt unless it reaches to a poisonous stage. Nature tries to give warnings in the form of headache, heat in the body, difficulty in passing stools, a slight pain in one of the limbs.

But when the trouble becomes unbearable, man goes to the doctor, who gives some medicines or injections, which stops the symptoms and pain for the time being. Again with slight excitement the diseases relapse in another form and man becomes a habitual sufferer. In this age of world-wide control, we have neither control over the causes leading to constipation, nor over the necessaries of daily life. We must seek ways and means to follow the current of circumstances and prevent ourselves from being swept away by the current of worldly affairs, as we cannot avoid the strain and stress of the present civilised life.

How to Prevent Constipation

Some such means may be followed as given below to prevent constipation:

1. Warm or cold bath should be taken early in the morning. Cold bath will be preferable.

2. A cup or two of cold water or warm water may be drunk in the morning.

3. Some exercises such as walking, running, trunk-bending, Asanas, Pranayama or deep breathing or other physical exercises should be performed daily either early in the morning or in the evening.

4. One should soak handful of wheat or any kind of grams in cold water in a cup over night and drink that liquid and eat those soaked articles, masticating them well in the mouth.

5. Urge to pass urine or faecal matters should not be curbed. Even the poorest of the poor beggars can follow the above means.

6. Middle class men can have a cycle ride instead of walking early in the morning and physical exercises which require some sort of apparatus.

7. Instead of grains soaked in water, they can take a

chhatak of Raisins, figs, or dates, soaked in water over night.

8. Instead of a mere cup of warm or cold water they can take water mixed with the juice of a lemon, orange or Mosambi.

9. They should take enema once in a week if they can afford and if it is possible in the poor accommodation, which is the lot of the middle class men.

10. Failing this they can take a teaspoonful senna leaves, soak them in a cup of cold water overnight and drink the liquid either warm or cold in the morning once in a week.

11. Occasional i.e. weekly or fortnightly fasts of 12 or 24 hours can be observed whenever and wherever possible. Because nowadays it becomes very difficult to observe a fast as too many shops of eatables can be found everywhere which tempt us very much.

12. Excess of tea, coffee, or cold drinks or other bazaar sweets should be avoided. For all these self-control is most necessary. It can be gained by reading religious books.

13. Possible Brahmacharya should be observed. Prayers should be offered to God *at least* early in the morning when you get up from the bed and when you go to bed, and God's Name should be repeated and remembered in the mind whenever and wherever possible.

14. Waking up late hours in the night should also be avoided.

15. Food should contain as much roughage as possible, but this is impossible now, as pounding and grinding is done by machines. In cities and towns it is not possible to grind grains at home because there is not enough space for lodging and many have to live in one room or in a congested space. So those who can afford should have 50% of cheap leafy green vegetables in their meals, but many

men cannot afford even vegetable, then what to say of milk and milk-products which have become a rarity in many homes.

16. Instead of vegetables, one can take leaves of Bael, sweet neem, but it is difficult to get these also in cities and towns.

If some of these rules are faithfully observed we can have ordinary health at least.

Chronic Constipation and Its Cure

Constipation if neglected in the beginning becomes chronic and troublesome in the long run. So I shall now suggest means to cure chronic constipation.

Remedies more effective, than medicines of any pathies, for permanent and lasting cure are (1) Fast, (2) Enema (3) Fruitarian diet.

Most persons hate fasts, so at least enema must be resorted to. Enema may be taken daily continuously for some days until there is normal movement of the bowels. As fasts are neither liked nor are suitable to many, at least one meal should consist of fruits or leafy vegetables.

Trunk bending exercises, some Asanas like Paschi-mottanasana, Bhujangasana, Mayurasana, Sarvangasana — should be performed.

As it is troublesome to take a hip or sitz bath daily, a cold water pack over the abdomen should be kept daily twice for at least 20 minutes each time. This will serve the purpose of a hip bath.

Cold water bath should be taken daily if it will agree to your constitution.

A cup of hot water should be tried half an hour to one hour before meals.

In each meal use a little ginger and salt before beginning your meals.

Instead of tea or coffee take juice of a lemon in a cup of warm water mixed with a little salt or sugar or honey, daily, according to your taste. A bread of coarse flour will not cause constipation.

All the remedies mentioned above have been tried, tested and found to be true and some of them are within the reach of even a poor man.

Fruits available in the season should invariably be taken as they give vitality and are nature's remedies.

A man suffering from constipation can take the following:

All leafy vegetables, cauliflower, tomatoes, carrots, fruits and pod vegetables, figs, dates, raisins, papaya.

Ganesh Kriya, i.e., inserting the finger in the anus and taking out faecal matter in the form of hard clogs, may also be used, whenever necessary.

Mud-plaster over the abdomen is beneficial. Put the plaster on the lower abdomen and cover it with a plantain leaf and bandage. Try this plaster patiently for some weeks. The plaster must be formed of plastic moist clay. Water should dribble from the plaster.

As for a medicine on constipation one is recommended to use Biochemic constipation Powder as Biochemic medicines are harmless and also much effective, and very convenient for administration.

Drugless Treatment of Constipation

1. **Ushapani Treatment:** Drink a tumbler of tepid or cold water in the early morning, and at night also. You can do also big sips of cold water 9 or 10 times in the early morning.

2. **Dietetic Treatment:** Take plenty of green vegetables, fruits, bael fruit, butter.

3. **Yogic Treatment:** Practise Asanas such as Sarvanga, Hala, Uttanapadasana, Paschimottanasana, Bhujangasana, Salabhasana, Nauli, Uddiyana, Agnisara, Suryanamaskar, Kumbhaka (Pranayama). Practise Ganesh Kriya if there is accumulation of faeces in the rectum.

4. **Hydropathic Treatment:** Take hip bath. Massage the abdomen.

5. **Colour Treatment:** Yellow is one of the healthiest colours. It is a laxative.

6. Massage the abdomen with a little sesamum or mustard oil. Massage round the navel in a clockwise manner.

7. Take enema if necessary.

Abdominal Massage

Abdominal massage stimulates circulation of blood and helps dislodgment of accumulated faecal matter.

The direction of the massage should be along the course of the large intestine. Start from the right lower corner across the top of the abdomen and down the left side to the left lower corner. This is one round. Repeat this several times. Use gingely or mustard oil for massage.

The direction of massaging the abdomen should be along the large bowel.

Massage gently, patiently and leisurely. Do not do it in a hurry. Massage must be comforting to the patient. Stop the massage when it becomes irksome and uncomfortable to the patient.

Massage with oil will supply nutrition to the patient. One or two ounces may be absorbed in this region alone in course of an hour.

Also massage around the navel clockwise.

Diet for Constipation
All-Fruit Diet
I

Live on all-fruit diet for one or two weeks. All-fruit diet is Nature's finest eliminating medium.

Fresh, juicy fruits fill the body with life-giving mineral salts, and cleanse the tissues. They overcome all diseased conditions. They are highly beneficial in chronic constipation.

II

Porridge, wholemeal bread, apples, figs, prunes, oranges, vegetables such as spinach, lady's finger, paraval, Methi, etc., are highly beneficial.

The diet should contain plenty of fruits and vegetables particularly salads and tomatoes. Oatmeal is a laxative.

III

Take such articles of food as leave a large-intestinal residue, such as coarse bread, bran bread containing bran, rice, oatmeal Porridge, fruits, especially bananas, vegetables, especially greens, in abundance, butter.

IV

1. Drink a tumbler of plain water, tepid or cold as the first thing in the morning, or eat an apple, pears, bunch of grapes, banana, orange etc.

2. Breakfast: Porridge, Bran, stewed prunes, wholemeal bread with plenty of butter, honey or treacle or well-cooked oatmeal with a little milk, Marmalade, (a jam or preserver generally made of the pulp of oranges, originally of quinces.)

3. Lunch: Vegetables, greens and salads wholemeal

bread and butter cream, cheese, fruits, cabbage, brussels sprouts, cauliflower, beans, carrots, stewed fruits, fruit pudding.

Dinner — Vegetable soup, vegetables, salads, fruits, whole-meal bread and butter, pudding. Fluids may be taken freely.

V

Fresh green vegetables such as lettuce, dried fruits such as raisins, and lemon juice, berries, rhubarb and sprouts are highly beneficial in chronic constipation.

Nature-Cure:

Here is the nature-cure for constipation.
Chew a few bael leaves
And sweet neem-leaves daily.
Eat ladies' finger, Paraval, Lauki, Spinach (Palak),
Drink water freely,
Take bael fruit, apples,
Fig, Prunes, tamarind-sherbet.
Date, Guava, honey.
Take hip-bath or sitz-bath.
Massage the abdomen nicely
Take a tumbler of water at night.
And in the early morning.
Imbibe yellow colour.
Do exercise regularly.

Biochemical Remedies for Constipation

Kali Mur. — Constipation with light coloured stools; white greyish-white coated tongue; fatty food and pastry disagree.

Natrum Mur. — Dryness of the bowels, with watery eyes, watery vomit. Dull, heavy headache; hard, dry stools difficult to pass; torn, smarting feeling after stool.

Natrum Sulph. – Hard, knotty, stools. sometimes streaked with blood. Difficult to expel soft stools.

Silicea – Faeces recede after being partly expelled. Constipation of poorly-nourished children.

Chapter XI

CHROMOPATHY

Chromopathic Cure for Constipation and Piles

The use of Sunlight and Colour for relieving and removing Constipation and Piles is a very simple, effective, pleasant and easy method of treatment. The distinctive, advantages of this mode of treatment is that it is readily available everywhere. There is sunlight to one and all without having the trouble of visiting the bazaar to purchase things and prepare medicines. It is absolutely free and thus open to the poorest, absolutely easy to make and pleasant to take. No bitter smell or taste to be tolerated by the patient and no unpleasant effects. Natural, simple, economical and clean is the chromopathic treatment. For the poorest, the most fastidious, and the delicate — to all this method is suitable.

Out of the colours Red, Yellow, Blue, Orange, Green, Violet and Purple, the two colours namely YELLOW and ORANGE are those useful in treating Constipation.

Yellow and Orange are gently stimulating and *laxative* in quality. They are laxative, purgative and stimulating to the bile.

These two colours help in overcoming constipation and remove effectively all sluggishness of liver and bowels. Water charged with Sun's rays through yellow coloured glass is an unfailing cathartic and in small doses is a gentle laxative. Such yellow water is also very good for treating Piles and Haemorrhoids.

How to Medicate: Clean glass bottles of the desired

colour to be used. Fill it three quarters with purest water. Rain water is best. If not pure, water well filtered several times will serve the purpose. Keep it exposed to the direct rays of the sun, the best time being between 11 a.m. to 3 p.m. Water or sugar thus medicated should not be exposed to other lights like moonlight, gas or electric light, lamp-light etc., etc.

For use during travelling and during rainy season sugar is an excellent medium for medication. It should be exposed 4 or 5 hours daily for about 4 weeks. Then it is ready for use and it also retains the effect for a considerable period. Thus its special use during rainy months when good sunlight may not be available for several days together.

Dosage and Administration: For Chromopathy water 1 ounce is the normal average dose for the adult. It may be taken twice daily early in the morning and at night when retiring to bed. In most cases this would suffice very well.

The medicated sugar may be administered in 4 to 5 grain doses for the normal adult. If frequent doses are necessary (as may be preferred in treating acute cases) about 20 grains of the Chromo-sugar may be mixed with about 3 to 4 ounces of water and a spoonful taken every hour.

Modes of treatment: Besides colour-charged water and sugar as mentioned above people with Piles and Constipation are benefited by including in their diet *Yellow* and *Orange* coloured fruits and vegetables. For instance ripe yellow mangoes, ripe papaya fruit, yellow plantains, yellow dates, yellow lemons, sweet limes, oranges, etc., are all excellent Nature's own ready-made Chromotheraphic agents.

The regular treatment by exposing the abdominal region to coloured sunlight passed through yellow glass pane is an auxiliary mode of treatment. The patient of Piles and Constipation may also wear yellow clothes for some time during the day where this is possible without embarrassment.

Chapter XII

HOMEOPATHIC TREATMENT OF CONSTIPATION

I

Natr. Mur. 6x 2h in hot water. Small frequent and unfinished stools Nux V. 30 4h. Stools large and hard as if burnt. Dryness of mouth. Bitter taste. Thirst. Bry. 30 4h. Constipation of bottle-fed babies even soft stool is passed with difficulty. Alumins 30 4h. Patient is afraid to sit for stools on account of pain during and after the stools Sulph 30 4h. With bleeding piles Collin 30 4h. No desire for stools for days Opium 5x 2h.

II

Aesculus 6-30 – Frequent ineffectual urging to stool (Nux.). Stools large, dry, hard, difficult to pass; rectum dry, hot and aching; *feels full of sticks.* Severe backache. Blind piles.

Alumen 30-200 – Obstinate constipation. No inclination to stool (Bry.), ineffectual urging (Nux), cannot expel stool. *Marble-like masses pass but rectum still feels full.* Itching pain and smarting of rectum after stool, Haemorrhoids.

Alumina 30-200 – Hard, dry, knotty stools, no desire (Bry.). Rectum sore, dry, inactive, even a *soft stool is passed with difficulty* (Stan). *Constipation of bottle-fed babies,* of infants; and of old persons (Lyco., Op.) or pregnant women (Collin., Sep.), from inactive rectum, *great straining, must grasp something tight.* Ailments from lead.

Byronia 6-30 – *Stools large, dry, hard, as if burnt; in hot weather,* after being heated. Feeling of a stone in the stomach; dry parched lips and mouth, great thirst; bitter taste; headache. *No desire for stools.* Inactivity of rectum.

Collinsonia 6-30 — Most obstinate *constipation with piles;* hard, dry stools. Sensation of *sharp sticks in the rectum.* Constipation of children and of pregnant women.

Lycopodium 30-200 — Ineffectual urging. Stool scanty, hard, passes with difficulty; after stool, sensation as if *much remained behind.* Sensation of fullness in the abdomen after a light meal. Loud rumbling and croaking in the *lower abdomen;* Excessive accumulation of wind; gastric derangements. *Belching gives no relief* (China). Painful piles, sensitive to touch, discharge of blood even with a soft stool.

Magnesia mur. 6-200 — Stool hard, scanty, large, knotty, like sheep-dung (Plumb.), difficult to pass. *Constipation of infants during dentition.* Painful Haemorrhoids.

Nux-vomica 30-200 — Frequent *ineffectual urging to stool;* passes but small quantity at a time. Stools incomplete and unsatisfactory, sensation as if part remained behind (Lyco.) Painful piles.

Opium 6-30 — Obstinate constipation, no desire for stool. *Stools, round, hard,* black. Stool comes out and goes back (Sil.). Abdomen hard, bloated and tympanitic.

Plumbum 6-30 — Constipation, may be with violent colic. Stools hard; small balls stuck together in a lump, difficult to pass; urging and painful spasm in anus. *Sheep-dung stools.* Excruciating pain or colic due to inflammation of the appendix.

Sepia 30-200 — Unsuccessful urging, sensation of a lump in rectum. Stool insufficient, hard, knotty, in balls like sheep-dung (Plumb.); stool mixed up or covered with mucus. Pain in rectum during and long after stool. Sense of weight in anus not relieved by evacuation. Discharge of blood with stool. Constipation with prolapsus of uterus. Constipation of pregnant women (Alumina).

Silicea 30-200 – *Constipation of women* especially *before and during menses.* Rectum feels inactive or paralysed. Stool comes down with difficult and much straining. *Stool goes back when partly expelled* (Thuja). *Fistula in ano.* Fissures and haemorrhoids.

Sulphur 30-200 – Stools large, hard, knotty, dry as if burnt (Bry.); insufficient, frequent ineffectual urging (Nux); very painful; *patient is afraid to have the stool* on account of pain. Redness around anus with itching. Piles. *Psoric constitution.*

Thuja 30-200 – Obstinate constipation ineffectual urging. Stool in hard balls. Stool goes back when partly expelled (Sil.), Haemorrhoids, *very painful.*

III

Constipation: In sedentary people, dark, spare; ineffectual urging; frequent desire, but only very little passes, *Nux v.* 1-30, 8h. After Nux. if this is insufficient; in persons who are subject to skin eruptions; who suffer from fainting spells, flushing of heat to the head, or sinking sensation at the pit of the stomach, especially about 11 a.m.; frequent ineffectual urging to stool, insufficient stool, sensation as if something remained behind in rectum, piles which bleed periodically, *Sul.* 3-30, 8h.

Torpor of bowels, stool hard, large, dry, Bry. 3, 6h.

Torpor of bowels; stool small, hard pieces like marbles; dark brown, with drowsiness, *OP.* 3, 6h.

Drowsiness, chillness, flatulence, *Nux mos.* 30, 6h.

Very obstinate constipation, dry lumpy stool painless, or with severe colic and retraction of abdomen, *Plumb. acet.* 3 gr.ii. 6, 6h.

Hard, scantily stool, painful in passing, burning in rectum, passage of blood, *Nit. ac.* 1, 4h.

Large, knotty stool, covered with white shreds of mucus, expelled with much effort; associated with delayed menses, *Graph.* 6, 6h.

Hard knotty stool, with or without blind piles, much pain in the back; sensation of fulness in rectum after stool; sensation in rectum as if full of small sticks, AEsc. h. 1, 6h.

Accumulation of faeces in rectum, *Chin.* 1, 2h.

Stool like sheep's dung; pain in region of liver, *magnes. mur.* 5, 6h.

Stool tough, shiny, knotty, like sheep's dung, oily; pressure in rectum as if faeces lodged in it, *Caust.* 5, gtt. ii. 4h.

Stool hard, small, dry crumbling, *Zinc. met.* 6, 4h.

Black, pitchy stool, *Zinc. mur. 3,* 4h.

Stool retained, sensation as if rough faeces remained in rectum, feeling of constriction at anus arresting it; especially in ill-nourished persons with unhealthy complexion: associated with deficient menses *Nat. m.3,* gr. ii. – 6, 6h

Slow, insufficient stool; sensation of weight or ball in anus not relieved by stool, *Sep.* 6, 4h.

With distention of the abdomen, flatulence passing downwards, water high-coloured, with deposit of lithates, hard difficult stool, *Lyc.* 6, 6h.

Dilated and paralysed rectum; lumpy stools, *Alumina,* 6, 6h.

Stools hard as stones; passes much blood; constipation of uterine or rectal cancer, *Alumen,* 30, 6h.

No desire for stool; constipation alternating with looseness of the bowels; constipation with dull headache;

after abuse of purgatives; with foul tongue; with piles, *Hydrast.* 1, 6h.

Stool difficult to pass on account of hardness and size, *Verat. a.* 3, 6h

Palliatives: A satisfactory evacuation can often be obtained by *Merc. dulc.* ix. gr. iii. 4h. for a few doses.

Persons who have been in the habit of taking purgatives and fear to leave them off *Sul.,* at bed-time.

A glass of cold water drunk, fasting will often suffice to ensure a good evacuation. Or a glass of cold water may be taken at bed-time; or, if cold water is not tolerated, hot water instead. Or this: a tablespoonful of coarse treacle put into a tumbler of water overnight, and drunk by sips in the morning whilst dressing.

In constipation in infants, manna used for sweetening their food is often of great service. If other things fail, *Hydrast,* gtt. iii. in a wine-glassful of water, taken in the morning fasting, acts as a mild aperient. A sitz-bath every second night (65 − 75 F.), for five or ten minutes, the body and limbs being kept thoroughly warm during the time, is often of great assistance where there is torpor of the bowels. A cold water or tepid water compress may be worn across the body at night.

Whenever constipation is one of many symptoms of disordered health, the medicines directed to the chief disorder will usually remove the constipation also: *Spigelia* in heart affections, *Iris* in migraine, *Gels.* in headaches.

IV

Obstinate followed by diarrhoea: stools,
   hard and clay-coloured   Nux V.   30
Sedentary people − 3ineffective urging
   after abuse of purgative   Nux V.   200
Subjected to skin affections   Sul.   30

After taking rich or fat food	Puls.	30
Due to train journey frequent urging	Plat	30
No desire for stool for days	Alum	30
Stools, hard, lumpy, black, of children with large bellies	Plumb	6
Knotty stools like sheep-dung	Caust	30
Of infants during teething, stools knotty	Magm	30
Persons subject to take much laxative	Hydr.	2X
In infants, pain sickly	Pso	30
In heart affections	S-pig	30
In headaches	Gles	30
Brown tongues, irritability, headache	Bry	30
Frequent ineffectual urging, restless sleep	Nux vom.	30
Tarpid bowels, hard and lumpy, retention of urine, drowsiness	Op.	30
Habitual constipation painful, distention of abdomen	Sul	6X

Chapter XIII

UNANI REMEDIES FOR CONSTIPATION

1. Apply castor oil on Betel leaf and warm a bit and put it on the abdomen of the child.

2. Heat a loaf on one side only, apply sesamum (til) oil on unheated side and put it on the abdomen of the child and bandage it.

3. Saunf, Ilaichi (big), Ajwain, Pudina (Mint), take distilled waters of all 4 medicines, mix them and heat a bit and take it in the morning.

4. Boil Saunf (dill seed) in water and drink it two or three times in a day.

5. Boil Banafsha (violet flowers) in milk and drink it.

6. Habitual constipation—Almonds 14, Gul banafsha 9 Mashas, Mazez Munaqqa 9, put all medicines in clean white piece of cloth and boil it in 12 oz, milk, when milk is reduced to half the quantity, remove the contents, clean through sieve or cloth, dissolve Misri to sweeten it and take it in the morning daily for a few days.

7. Sanna makki 1½ tola, Nasout Mudabbar 3¾ Mashas, Gul Gulab 4½ Mashas, mix and powder them fine, take with hot water in the morning.

8. Turbad white one tola, Anisun 7 Mashas, Sanna makki 7 Mashas, Gul sukh 5 Mashas, Asara Revand 2 Mashas, Hub ulnil 6 Mashas, Ilaichi white 3 Mashas, Ailwa 3 Mashas, Post Halela Zard 3 Mashas, Zira white 3 Mashas, powder them fine. Dose 1½ Mashas in the night with cow's milk.

9. Sabar Siah 6 Mashas, Asara Revand 6 Mashas, Hub

ulnil one tola, mix all of them and prepare pills in water; take 3 pills with hot water or milk in the morning.

10. Atraifal Zaman, Atraifal Sannai or Atraifal Mullain, take any one, one tola with milk at night only.

11. Gulkand 2 tolas or 2 pieces of Har ka Murabba with milk at night.

12. Har, Bahera, Amla, Sounth, Kali Mirch, and Pipal — 6 Mashas each; powder them fine and take 3 Mashas powder with cold water.

13. Nashaunth 3 tolas, Triphala 3 tolas, Bhibarang one tola, Pipal one tola, Joakhar one tola, Gur one year old 3 tolas; prepare pills of 6 Mashas each; one pill with hot water.

Chapter XIV

YOGIC PANACEA FOR CONSTIPATION

Yogic exercises are preservative and curative. That is the beauty of this system. Some exercises twist the body forward and backward. Others help the lateral movements of the spine. Thus the body as a whole is developed, toned up and strengthened.

Yoga Asanas are intended for the thorough exercise of the internal organs, viz., liver, spleen, pancreas, intestines, heart, lungs, brain and the important ductless glands of the body which are called endocrine glands, viz., thyroid and parathyroid at the root of the neck, adrenals in spleen pituitary and pineal glands in brain which play a very important part in the economy of nature, in maintaining health in metabolism and in structure, growth and different kinds of cells and tissues of the nutrition of body.

The diaphragm, the muscular partition between the chest and the abdomen is also developed by certain exercises such as Dhanurasana, Mayurasana, Paschimottanasana. The movements of the diaphragm massage the abdominal viscera or organs. There will be free evacuation of the bowels daily in the morning. Constipation, dyspepsia and a host of other ailments of the stomach and the intestines will be eradicated.

The whole course of Yoga Asanas can be finished in fifteen minutes. Within this short period you can realise the maximum benefit. All the organs of the body are toned up and exercised. This system is simple, exact efficacious, economical of time and capable of being self-practised.

Here are a few Asanas which if practised cure all cases of constipation.

Sarvangasana: This in one of the unique poses which rejuvenates the whole system.

Technique: Spread a thick blanket on the ground. Lie quite flat on the back. Slowly raise the legs. Lift the trunk, hips and legs quite vertical. Rest the elbows on the ground firmly and support the back with the two hands. Raise the legs till they become quite vertical. Press the chin against the chest. This is the chin-lock. While you perform this Asana the back of the neck, the posterior part of the head and the shoulders should touch the ground. Breathe slowly and concentrate on the thyroid glands which are situated in the neck. Do not allow the body to shake to and fro. When the Asana is over, lower the legs very slowly and with elegance. Avoid jerks. Do the Asana very gracefully. In this Asana the whole weight of the body is thrown on the shoulders. You can do this Asana twice daily, morning and evening. Immediately after performing this Asana, you will have to do Matsyasana to derive the full benefit from it. Remain in this Asana for two minutes and gradually increase the period to 30 minutes.

This easy and wonderful Asana is intended to promote the secretion of the thyroids and through it the whole body and all its functions. The thyroids are the most important glands of the endocrine system. In this Asana the thyroid glands receive a rich supply of blood. Healthy thyroids mean healthy functioning of the circulatory, respiratory, alimentary and genito-urinary systems of the body.

This Asana is a good substitute for modern thyroid treatment. It cures the dreadful leprosy. The patient will have to live on milk during the whole period of treatment. Milk helps the thyroid to secrete its juice in sufficient quantity to help the economy of nature in its restorative function and regeneration. If the patient takes a sun-bath morning and evening, his recovery will be hastened.

This Asana keeps back the ravages of old age and keeps a man young always. Those young men who have lost weight of the testes owing to bad habits like masturbation, sexual excesses, etc., will retain the weight by this Asana. They can combine Uddiyana Bandha and Nauli Kriya and regain their lost vitality and energy.

Sarvangasana cures dyspepsia, constipation, appendicitis, other gastro-intestinal disorders and varicose-veins. It supplies a large quantity of blood to the spinal roots of the nerves. It is this Asana which centralises the blood in the spinal column and nourishes it beneficially. Except through this Asana, the nerve roots cannot receive an adequate blood supply. It keeps the spine quite elastic. Elasticity of the spine means everlasting youth. It prevents the bone from early ossification (hardening). Sarvangasana awakens Kundalini and augments the digestive power.

Halasana: On completion, this pose gives the exact appearance of a plough. Hala means a 'plough'.

Lie flat on your back on a carpet. Keep the two hands near thighs, the palms towards the ground. Without bending the legs slowly raise them higher up. Do not raise the hands but raise the hips and the lumbar part of the back also and bring down the legs till the toes touch the ground beyond the head. Keep the knees quite straight and close together. The legs and thighs must be in one straight line. Press the chin against the chest. Breathe slowly through the nose. This is Sarvangasana. Remain in this Asana for two minutes. Then slowly raise the legs and bring them to the original position of lying on the ground flat.

There is a better variety of this Asana. When the toes reach the ground, remove the hands and catch hold of the toes. The pose can be repeated 3 to 6 times with advantage. For attaining spiritual benefits, the pose should be maintained for a long time at a stretch.

Benefits: In Bhujanga, Salabha and Dhanurasana the deep and superficial muscles of the back are contracted and relaxed, but in Halasana these muscles are fully stretched and relaxed. These muscles of the back are responsible for the healthy condition of the spine. The abdominal muscles contract vigorously and become very strong. The whole spine is steadily pulled posteriorly. Every vertebrae and ligament that is attached to it receive plenty of blood and become healthy. All the 31 pairs of spinal nerves and the sympathetic system are well nourished by a copious blood supply and so are toned up. This Asana prevents the early ossification of the vertebral bones. He who practises this Asana is very nimble, agile and full of energy. Various sorts of myalgia, lumbago, sprain in the neck, neuralgia, etc., are cured. Obesity or corpulence and habitual or chronic constipation, gulma (chronic dyspepsia), liver and spleen complaints are also cured.

Bhujangasana: When this Asana is fully done, it gives the appearance of a hooded cobra. The raised trunk, neck and head represent the hood. Hence the significant name. 'Bhujanga' means a cobra in Sanskrit.

Technique: Lie down on the blanket keeping the back above. Relax all the muscles completely. Place the palms below the corresponding shoulders on the blanket. Raise the head and upper portion of the body slowly just as the cobra raises its hood. Bend the spine well. Do not raise the body — suddenly with a jerk. Raise it little by little so that

/ou can actually feel the bending of the vertebrae one by one and the pressure travelling downwards from the cervical, dorsal and lumber regions and lastly to the sacral regions. Let the body from the navel downwards to the toes touch the ground. Retain the posture for a minute and slowly bring down the head little by little. You may repeat the process 6 times.

Benefits: All the Western physical culturists unanimously acclaim the importance of rendering the spine supple and elastic. Elasticity of the spine means health, vitality and youth to the individual. The deep and superficial muscles of the back are well toned up. This pose relieves the pain in the back that may have been caused due to overwork. The abdominal muscles are pulled and thereby strengthened. The intra-abdominal pressure is increased to a very high degree and so constipation is removed. The whole abdominal viscera are toned up. Every vertebrae and its ligaments are pulled backwards and they get a rich blood supply. It increases bodily heat and destroys a host of ailments. It gives good appetite.

Bhujangasana is particularly useful for ladies in toning up their ovaries and uterus. It is a powerful tonic. It will relieve amenorrhoea, dysmenorrhoea, leucorrhoea and various other utero-ovarine troubles.

Mayurasana: In Sanskrit "Mayur" means peacock. When this Asana is exhibited the body resembles a peacock which has spread out its bundle of feathers at the back.

Technique: Kneel on blanket. Join the two arms together and rest them on the ground, palms turned down. You may curve the fingers slightly. This facilitates balancing. Keep the hands firm. Now you have steady and firm forearms for supporting the whole body. Bring down the abdomen slowly against the conjoined elbows. Support your body on your elbows. Then stretch your legs. Inhale and raise the legs together from the ground. Raise the legs straight on a level with the head, parallel to the ground. Keep the posture steady for five seconds and then rest the toes on the ground and exhale. This is Mayurasana. Rest for a few minutes.

Benefits: This is the best Asana known for all stomach disorders. Owing to the pressure of hands on the stomach below the navel, the abdominal aorta is partially compressed and the blood that is thus checked is directed towards the digestive organs. The liver, pancreas, stomach, kidneys are toned up. The intra-abdominal pressure is increased to a very high degree and the abdominal viscera is toned up. Mayurasana awakens the Kundalini Shakti.

Mayurasana has got a charm of its own. It braces you up quickly. It serves like a hypodermic injection of adrenaline or digitalin. This is a wonderful Asana for improving digestion. Sluggishness of the liver or hepatic torpidity disappears. This one Asana can give you maximum benefit in a minimum space of time; a few seconds daily are enough.

Uddiyana Bandha: Empty the lungs by a strong and forcible expiration. Now contract and forcibly draw up the intestines and also the navel towards the back, so that the abdomen rests against the back of the body high up in the thoracic cavity. He who practises this Bandha constantly conquers death and becomes young. This helps a lot in keeping up Brahmacharya. Uddiyana Bandha is practised during Rechaka and at the end of Rechaka (exhalation). Uddiyana can be done in a sitting or a standing posture. When you practise this in the standing posture, place your hands on the thighs. Keep the legs apart and bend your trunk slightly.

Uddiyana Bandha imparts good health, strength, vigour and vitality to the practitioner. When it is combined with Nauli Kriya which consists in churning the abdomen, it serves as a powerful gastro-intestinal tonic. Uddiyana Bandha and Nauli Kriya are two potent weapons of the Yogi for combating against constipation, weak peristalsis of the intestines and the gastro-intestinal disorders of the alimentary system.

Nauli Kriya: Nauli Kriya is intended for regenerating, invigorating and stimulating the abdominal viscera and the gastro-intestinal or alimentary system. For the practice of Nauli, you should know Uddiyana Bandha well. Uddiyana Bandha can be done even in a sitting posture; but Nauli should be done only while standing.

Expire forcibly through the mouth and so keep the lungs completely empty. Contract and forcibly draw the abdominal muscles towards the back. This is Uddiyana Bandha.

For practising Nauli, stand up. Keep the right leg a foot apart from the left leg. Rest your hands on the thighs. Slightly bend forward. Then do Uddiyana Bandha. Now allow the centre of the abdomen to be free by contracting the left and right side of the abdomen. You will have all the muscles in the centre in a vertical line. This is Madhyama Nauli.

Contract the right side of the abdomen and allow the left side to be free. You will have all the muscles on the left side only. This is Vama Nauli. Again contract the left side muscles and allow the right side to be free. This is Dakshina Nauli. By carrying out such graduated exercises you will understand how to contract the muscles of the central, left and right side of the abdominal muscles. You will also notice how they move from side to side. In this stage you will see the abdominal muscles only in the central, the right or on the left side.

Keep the muscles in the centre. Slowly bring them to the right side and then to the left side in a circular way. Do this several times from right to left and then do it in a reverse way from the left to the right side. When you advance, you may do these more quickly. This last stage of Nauli will appear like 'churning' when the abdominal muscles are isolated and rotated from side to side.

When Nauli is demonstrated by advanced students, the onlookers will be extremely surprised to see the movements of the abdominal muscles. They will feel as if an engine was working in the abdominal factory. Those who have a tender body, can very easily learn and perform this Kriya in a beautiful and efficient manner.

Nauli Kriya eradicates chronic constipation, dyspepsia and all other diseases of the gastro-intestinal system. The liver and pancreas are toned up. The kidneys and the other organs of the abdomen are also made to function properly.

Salabhasana: "Salabha" means a 'locust' in Sanskrit. When the pose is demonstrated, it gives the appearance of a locust with its tail raised.

Technique: Lie prone (on the face) on the blanket and keep the hands alongside the body, palms facing upwards. Rest the chin on the ground by raising the head a little higher up or rest the chin, the mouth and the nose on the ground. Now inhale slowly. Stiffen the whole body and raise the legs high. The knees should be kept straight. The sacrum too should be raised a little along with the legs. Keep the thighs, legs and toes in a straight line. Remain in the pose for 20 seconds and slowly bring down the legs, and then exhale slowly. Repeat the process 3 or 4 times according to your capacity. Do not go so far as to induce fatigue. Bhujangasana exercises the upper part of the body and Salabhasana the lower extremity of the body.

Benefits: The intra-abdominal pressure is increased to a very high degree. It relieves constipation and tones up the liver, pancreas and kidneys. All the abdominal muscles are strengthened to a very great degree. The vertebrae of the lumbar and the sacrum bone also get toned up. The sacral, coccygeal and the lower part of the lumber regions receive plenty of blood and so become healthy and strong. Owing to the Kumbhaka done during this pose, the lungs expand and become strong.

Dhanurasana: When this Asana is performed, it gives the appearance of a bow. Dhanur means a bow. The stretched hands and legs represent the string of a bow; and the body and the thighs represent the bow proper.

Technique: Lie prone on the blanket. Relax the muscles. Now bend the legs over the thighs. Catch hold of the right ankle with the right hand the left ankle with the left hand firmly. Raise the head, body and the knees by tugging at the legs with the hands so that the whole burden of the body rests on the abdomen and the spine is nicely arched backwards like a bow.

Maintain this pose for a few seconds and then relax the body. You can either make a Kumbhaka or breaths normally. Even weak persons can do this Asana; a sudden movement of the body is required. Be steady. Do not jerk the body.

Dhanurasana complements or supplements Bhujang-asana. We can say it is a combination of Bhujanga and Salabhasana with the addition of catching the ankles. Bhujanga, Salabha and Dhanur Asanas form a valuable combination. They always go together. They form one set of Asanas. Dhanurasana should be repeated 3 or 4 times.

Benefits: The very appearance of the pose gives one the idea that it is a combination of Bhujangasana and Salabhasana. All the benefits of Salabha and Bhujangasanas can be derived to a greater degree in Dhanurasana. The back muscles are well massaged. This removes constipation and cures dyspepsia, rheumatism and gastro-intestinal disorders. It reduces fat, energises digestion, invigorates appetite and relieves congestion of the blood in the abdominal viscera. This Asana is highly suitable for ladies.

Chapter XV

YOGA THERAPY

Sit on Padma, Siddha or Sukha Asana.
Close your eyes.
Chant OM six times.
Go through any anatomical or physiological book.
Look at the bowel-picture very carefully.
Now concentrate on the bowels.
Have a picture of the bowels before the mind's eye.
Feel that the peristalsis is going on vigorously.
Again and again repeat this feeling.
Start it from the caecum.
Let it move through the ascending,
Transverse, descending colons.
Sigmoid flexure and rectum.
Now you will get up
To answer the calls of Nature.
This is an effective method.

Ganesh Kriya

If there are very hard lumps of faecal matter near the anus, no purgatives or enema can remove them. These Scybalae or hard lumps are like big corks.

In such cases the Ganesh Kriya should be practised. As Lord Ganesh is the presiding deity of the Muladhara Chakra near the anus, this Kriya is known as Ganesh Kriya.

Lubricate your left middle finger with any oil. Introduce it into the anus and remove the hard lumps slowly. This is Ganesh Kriya.

Constipation's Soliloquy

Oh! what a sad state of affairs, now!
I was once a king of all diseases.
I was the root or source of all maladies.
I induced faecal toxaemia.
I made millions my victims.
I attacked gentlemen with sedentary habits
And ladies with light corsets.
I assumed various forms,
Acute, chronic, habitual, occasional.
Sometimes I plugged the anus with scybalae.
No enema, no suppository, no purgative
Can come near me.
I am now terribly afraid of Sivananda.
He has taught Ganesh Kriya, Nauli and
Yoga Asanas to all people.
His book on constipation has revealed many secrets.
I am gone, I am gone for ever.
O am gone, I am gone for ever.
I have done my work efficiently here.
Salutations, O Mother dear, save me.

Chapter XVI

PILES SAQUELAE

(Haemorrhoids)

Causes, Symptoms and Treatment

I

Piles are swellings made up of blood vessels inside or around the margin of the anus. These swellings are caused by the dilatation or enlargement of the blood vessels in the terminating portion of the large bowel which is due to the stagnation of blood. The stagnation is produced by pressure as in the case of patients suffering from habitual constipation. The accumulated faecal matter presses upon the blood vessels continuously and as a consequence, they get dilated.

II

What are the causes, then, that lead on to this dire malady? They are: high living, habitual constipation, sedentary habits or avocations, riding, cycling, jolting in the case of persons whose pursuits engage them in constant cart journey, and abuse of strong purgatives.

III

In the beginning, the piles protrude while answering the calls of nature and at first go back spontaneously. Sometimes, they have to be replaced by the fingers. Later on protrusion of piles occurs at times other than during defaecation, and in protracted cases, they remain constantly protruded. At first, the motions are streaked with blood; but later on there is heavy loss of blood which makes the patient quite pale. The irritation and pain about the anus causes much annoyance.

IV

(a) The main element in the successful treatment of piles is that, in the first place, measures should be directed to combat against constipation. To have this desired effect, only *laxatives* which are extremely mild purgatives, should be selected.

(b) The parts around the anus should be kept scrupulously clean.

(c) Coffee and chillies which are irritants must be avoided. The diet should be quite bland and of a soothing nature.

(d) A large quantity of onions may be taken during supper. Onions contain a large amount of sulphur which exerts a beneficial influence.

(e) A small amount of castor oil or one or two plantain fruits may be taken with much advantage at bed time.

1. Confection of Sulphur   drachm 1
   To be taken three times a day.

2. Compound Liquorice powder
   only at bed time.   drachms 2

3. Gall & Opium ointment or conium ointment should be applied locally around the anus.

4. Hazeline cream, if applied, stops bleeding immediately with great efficacy.

But, above all, the radical treatment lies in removing the piles by having recourse to proper surgical and when palliative measures after a fair trail have proved of no avail.

Chapter XVII

STORY OF PILES

The other name for Piles is Haemorrhoids. The Sanskrit name is Arsa. The Hindi name is Bhavaseer.

Piles is a varicose condition of the rectal veins. Piles are swellings inside or around the margin of the anus, the terminal opening of the alimentary canal, the result of a varicose state of blood vessels.

The most common of all diseases of the anus is piles. There are two varieties of piles, internal and external. The internal variety lies under the anal canal. It cannot be seen from the outside unless they are prolapsed. The external variety lies outside, just at the place where the skin joins the lining of the end of the bowel. Each pile consists of a little bunch of varicose veins.

The piles may be partly internal and partly external. Internal piles may in some cases be seen, when the patient bears down, as purple swellings just protruding from the sphincter. In other cases piles are discovered only on digital examination of the rectum. In digital examination the finger is introduced into the rectum.

Examination may be conducted by passing the lubricated finger inside the rectum. The patient lies on his left side with the right thigh drawn up.

The rectum is a terminal point where a large number of veins or arteries meet. It is so situated that blood has to travel up against gravity. If there is congestion or obstruction in any of the organs placed above, stagnation is liable to occur. Diseases of the liver heart disease, obstinate habitual constipation etc., are causes of the disease.

Symptoms: Streaks of bright red blood occur in the motions. Sometimes even 4 pints of blood may be passed at one time.

There is pain during answering calls of nature. The pain continues for some time after the passage of a motion. When a pile becomes inflamed or strangulated by the sphincter, there are great pain and discomfort. The patient may have to remain in bed for days. Pain may be referred to other parts of the body — e.g., to the testicles, bladder, or loins.

Constipation always accompanies piles due partly to mechanical obstruction and partly to the pain caused by defaecation.

In several cases there are constitutional symptoms such as lassitude, irritability. headache, faintness and anaemia or poverty of blood from loss of blood.

Causes: (1) Portal obstruction is itself cause of piles.

(2) Habitual constipation is doubtless the most common cause of piles, particularly in women.

(3) Alcohol causes portal congestion and this becomes a source of piles. Alcohol in any form aggravates the condition.

(4) Sedentary occupation and deficient exercises also cause piles.

(5) Various local conditions such as sitting on soft cushions which construct the inferior haemorrhoidal veins, uterine displacements, pelvic and other tumours are all potent causes of piles.

In external piles a vein at the end of the anus gets enlarged and appears as a dark coloured tender smelling about the size of a pea. The swelling vanishes after some time. Some thickening is left on the skin. There spots are very tender and cause intense pain while answering the calls of nature. The external piles rarely bleed.

The internal piles bleed profusely. The bleeding occurs at the time of passing motions. The bleeding makes the person weak and anaemic. The internal piles may ulcerate and suppurate.

Piles are not usually regarded as serious, but they may be extremely troublesome by the constant loss of blood, by the pain they cause and by their liability to repeated attacks of inflammation.

The piles inside may prolapse. It is easy to replace to begin with but later on reduction becomes very difficult. It cannot get back. It becomes highly squeezed by the muscle around the anus. It gets inflamed and ulcerated.

Treatment: Find out the causes of piles and remove it.

Give up alcohol especially malt liquors and sugar.

Keep the piles scrupulously clean.

Replace the prolapsed piles at once.

Avoid rich food, wines and other causes of hepatic congestion.

Wash the part nicely after answering the calls of nature. Do not use toilet paper.

Repeated hot hip baths give great relief. Chloreton ointment, gall and opium ointment, conium ointment, Hamamelis with conium, morphia or cocaine are highly beneficial.

Confection of sulphur or confection of senna at night is very useful.

Paraffin is apt to cause the piles to descend.

Liquid Hazeline is excellent and is best applied on a piece of lint inserted with the anus and left there.

Myrobalan gives soft motions. The prolonged use of this medicine produces no evil effect. Obstinate piles may produce fissure and ulcer of the anus.

Take rest in bed when there is bleeding and inflammation.

Take very simple diet without spices. Take green vegetables and fruits.

Excessive bleeding may be stopped by application of ice cold water in a jet. Application of alum water, teaspoonful to 4 ounces of water will harden the surface and will have a healing effect.

A suppository containing 3 grains of Hamamelis and morphine for gr. $\frac{1}{8}$ is useful. It will remove pain and stop bleeding.

Inflamed piles are very painful. They are best treated by warm hip baths, warm fomentation with opium, belladonna or cocaine.

Inject the piles with 5 to 10 drops of 1 in 20 carbolic acid. Inject the fluid with a hypodermic needle into the centre of the pile. Thrombosis is caused and healing takes place by scar. The injected fluid makes the pile shrink until it practically disappears and bleeding stops at once. This is a satisfactory method of treatment. The injection is not painful. When this treatment is being carried out, the patient need not reduce his normal activities.

A strangulated pile may be incised radially under local anaesthesia and the clot removed.

Many cures are obtained by local high frequency and diathermy.

Boil 3 myrobalans in water. Add a drachm of alum to

decoction to make the lotion more astringent. Apply this lotion to the piles.

Make a paste of myrobalan (teaspoonful) and add 5 grains of opium. This will soothe the pain and irritation. Apply this to the piles.

Have an action of the bowels daily. Take the help of olive oil, medicinal paraffin if it is necessary. Take plenty of green vegetables, fruits, stewed fruits, etc.

If all these remedies fail, take recourse to surgical operation.

Improvement of general health and observance of rules of health and hygiene a long way towards healing piles.

Chapter XVIII

HINTS ON TREATMENT OF PILES

I

Piles is caused mainly by constipation, hard bowels or heat in the constitution.

Remove constipation. Drink plenty of water. Use enema or castophene pills or castor oil occasionally to keep bowels clean.

Perform the following Asanas: Paschimottanasana, Padahasthasana, Bhujangasana, Sarvangasana, Sirshasana, Siddhasana, Maha Mudra and Mula Bandha are highly effective.

Avoid all foodstuffs that irritate the bowels, pickles, spiced articles and condiments, chutneys and chillies, alcohol, too much sugar, and all kinds of rich and constipating foods.

Take vegetables especially the leafy ones, butter, especially acid fruits. Papaya is good.

Take hip bath for ten minutes daily.

Chandraprabha is an excellent specific especially in advanced cases of piles.

Take plenty of exercise. Long, brisk evening walks are excellent. Abdominal massage is very beneficial.

Treatment: For one week give 1 oz. of juice of raddish leaves with a little ghee. Peyampalam (a variety of plantain fruit available in Madras) soaked in castor oil and sugarcandy can be kept in a bottle and given daily, 2 spoonfuls with milk.

Inject into the rectum with a syringe one teaspoon of lemon juice mixed in four teaspoonfuls of sweet oil or water (or olive oil) at bed-time.

Alum water stops bleeding. Apply two or three days in a week.

Regulate your habits of life. Do regular Japa, Kirtan and meditation. Do not worry about the piles. Do Pranayama every morning. Feel that the Lord's Grace is flowing into you and curing you of the piles.

II

"From Ambrosia"

Bleeding Piles

Avoid constipation by tabloids of CASCARA SAGRADA invaluable for use in chronic constipation or CHELSEA PENSINOR or lenitive electuary (confection of sulphur and senna). Treat the cause; if not costiveness it may be due to sluggish liver, pressure in pelvis, stricture, tight belt, etc. Locally apply HAZELINE CREAM or COCAINE or EUCAINE in a lanoline and insert per rectum an enule suppository of gall and opium or tannic acid 3 grains with morphia ½ grain (half grain) twice a week.

Piles

The only way to get over the complaint radically is to undergo an operation and it is for yourself to decide whether the trouble is serious enough for such a course to be adopted. If not, continue the use of opium suppository when and as often as necessary. You would be better without alcohol entirely.

1. Nimbadi Kwath

Re: Daru Haldi (powder)   20 Tolas.
    Khas (powder)   20 Tolas.
    Outer Skin of Neem Tree (powder)   40 Tolas.

Mix well and strain. Add 8 seers of water to this. Boil down to a quarter. Filter the decoction. It can be preserved in the bottle for some time.

Take 2½ Tolas or 1 ounce every morning. Take this for 15 days.

2. Chitrakadi Choorna

Re: Chitrak Powder	7 Tolas
Hawoobair Powder	7 Tolas
Hing Powder	7 Tolas
Salt Powder (Sendha) Nimak	7 Tolas

Mix well and strain. Take 2 Tolas of the powder every morning with fresh butter milk.

3. Chitrakadi Dugdha (for bleeding piles)

Re: Lajvanti powder	2 Tolas
Mochrah Powder	2 Tolas
Kamal Kaisar	2 Tolas
Lodhra	2 Tolas
Rakta Chandan	2 Tolas
Chitrak	2 Tolas

Mix well. Boil it in half-a-seer of goat's milk till it is reduced to three-fourth. Strain the decoction and keep in a clean and tinned vessel.

Take 10 Tolas thrice daily in empty stomach.

4. Madhuparka Yoga

Re: Sonth Powder	½ Tola
Sugandhawala powder	½ Tola

Mix well and strain. Add 2 Tolas of good honey and 5 Tolas of raw rice water to 1 Tola of the above powder. (This is for one time).

Take before sunrise and after sunset. Do not take Jaggery, oil preparations, chillies and tamarind.

5. Kaisar Choorna I

Re: Black Til   2 Tolas
    Nag Kesar   2 Tolas
    Misri   2 Tolas

Powder these three and strain. Take one Tola of this powder with 2 Tolas of fresh butter in the early morning and at bed-time.

6. Rasanjan Yoga.

Re: Rasanjan Powder   2 Tolas
    Atis (Aconitun Heterophyllum)   2 Tolas
    Indra Jaun   2 Tolas

Make these three into fine powder and strain. Take one Tola of this powder and add to 5 Tolas or raw rice-water together with 2 Tolas of good honey. It is to be taken in the early morning for 15 days.

7. Kaisar Choorna II

Re: Misri (Sugar Candy)   3 Tolas
    Nag Kesar   3 Tolas

Make these two into powder. Take slight purgative before you take this medicine. One Tola of the above powder, may be mixed with 2 Tolas of fresh butter. One course is for eight days.

8. Aja Dugdha Yoga

Take goat's milk every day. It is also effective in piles.

9. Karela Rasa Yoga

Re: Extract 5 Tolas of juice from the green leaves of Karela creeper. Take 2 Tolas of sugar-candy and stir well the juice. Drink in the early morning. This is very effective in bleeding Piles.

10. Sooran Vati

Take 5 Tolas of Jimikand. Remove its outer skin and cut the rest into small bits as big as a gram. Put those bits in

sun for drying. Let them be dried nicely. After that cover
every bit of the above with half-a Tola of jaggery and put
them in the sun.

Take one tablet in the morning and one in the evening
with the water. One course is for 15 days.

11. Vidhaaraa Modak

Re: Vidhaaraa powder   4 Tolas
    Shuddha Bhilaava Powder   4 Tolas
    Sonth Powder   4 Tolas

Strain well. Boil 12 Tolas of sugarcandy (as confectioners
do) in a little water. Mix the powder well in the
sugarcandy-water. Let it become cold. Prepare Laddus
(balls) weighing 1 Tola each.

Take one Laddu (Ball) every day morning with cold
water.

Piles

1. Devadaalyaadi Lepa

Re: Vandaal seeds   5 Tolas
    Saindhava Namak (Salt)   5 Tolas

Grind these two and add fresh buttermilk to it, till an
ointment is prepared. Apply it to the anus, about one Tola
after answering the calls of nature.

2. Arshakuthaar Lepa

Re: Haridra Pushpa (flower)   2½ Tolas
    Shankha Choorna   2½ Tolas
    Mainasil   2 Tolas

Powder these three and add 10 Tolas of extract of Gaja
Pippali. Stir well till it becomes as thick as butter. Preserve
it in bottles. Apply to the rectum everyday.

3. Durnaphar Lepa

Re: Seeds of bitter Tumbi   5 Tolas
    Jaggery   2½ Tolas

Powder it and add to the fresh buttermilk, till it becomes an ointment. Apply this 2 to 3 times daily.

4. Ksheeraadi Lepa

Re: Arka Dugdha   2 Tolas
    Thohar Dugdha   2 Tolas
    Leaves of bitter Tumbi   2 Tolas
    Buds of Karanja   2 Tolas

Grind well. Prepare an ointment by mixing this to 10 Tolas of Goat's Urine. Apply this twice, morning and evening about ½ Tola of this ointment.

5. Shigru Mooladi Lepa

Re: Bark of the root of Suhaajan   3 Tolas
    Arka Patra   3 Tolas

Grind well in goat's milk and prepare ointment. Apply 8 to 4 times-a-day.

6. Akaachanfe Lepa

Re: Haridra   2 Tolas
    Bitter Turayee   2 Tolas

Grind well in 4 Tolas of mustard oil, till it becomes an ointment. Apply 1 Tola of this after answering the calls of nature.

7. Nimbaadi Lepa

Re: Neem leaves   2½ Tolas
    Kaneer leaves   2½ Tolas

Grind well and make it an ointment in 5 Tolas of butter milk. Apply twice-a-day.

8. Turaaksheeree Lepa

Re: Vanshalochan   1½ Tolas

Chotee Ilaayachee	1½ Tolas
Kattcha (Khadir Sattwa)	1½ Tolas
Neela Tootia (copper-sulphate)	1½ Tolas

Powder well. Stir well in lemon juice and make pills of 1 Tola. Dry the pills. Grind again each of the pill in water and apply 3 to 4 times daily.

9. Kaisaraadi Lepa

Re: Chotee Pippali	1 Tola
Haridra	1 Tola
Sankha Bhasma	½ Tola
Sazzi Kshaar	½ Tola
Leaves and seed of Karanjee	2 Tolas
Saindhava Namak (Salt)	1 Tola
Naag-kesar	2 Tolas
Ajwain	2 Tolas

Powder well and strain well through a cloth. Extract 15 Tolas of milk out of Arka leaves and grind the above powder with it. Dry the powder. Again stir well in cow's milk. Preserve it in bottles. Apply before sunrise and before going to the bed (to the rectum). Avoid oily preparations, chillies, tamarind, jaggery.

10. Ahiphenaadi Kalka

| Re: Nootan Bhang (fresh Bhang) | 1 Tola |
| Ahiphena | 1/12 Tola |

Powder in fresh water and make into poultice. Apply this to a piece of cloth. Heat it a little, and then tie it to the anus.

11. Guggalaadi Kalka

Re: Sugar-cane juice	½ Seer
Gingily Oil	2 Chattack
Suddha Guggul	5 Tolas

(a) Extract sugar-cane juice, first; (b) add this to ten

Tolas of gingily oil (c) boil it in low fire, till the oil alone remains and take it away from the fire; (d) take 5 Tolas of Guggul and strain it in 5 Tolas of milk. (e) Add this to the previous one, i.e., the boiled oil, till it becomes an ointment. Preserve it in tinned vessel. Apply 1 Tola every night before retiring to bed.

Biochemical Treatment

Calcar Flour – Principal remedy alternate with remedies for colour of tongue and blood. Bleeding piles with pressure of blood to the head. Pains low down in the back; chronically constipated.

Ferrum Phos. – Piles, with discharge of bright red blood, coagulating easily.

Natrum Sulph. – Piles, with much heat in the lower bowel, and associated with bilious conditions.

Magnesia Phos. – Pains in piles, of an acute, cutting, darting nature.

Kali Mur. – When the blood discharged is dark and thick.

Calcar Phos. – Intercurrently in piles of anaemic persons.

Natrum Mur. – Alternate with *Calcar Flour,* when stools are hard, dry and crumbling, with excess of saliva in the mouth.

External treatment: Use Calcar Flour, 2x, or 3x, and other remedies in solution or as ointment with vaseline.

Homeopathic Prescriptions for Piles

Blind piles in persons of sedentary life, spare, of the habit of having the motion of the bowels too slow Nux v. 3, 8h.

Bleeding piles, costiveness, sinking at the stomach,

especially in the forenoon; flushing; fainty spells; heat of the head with cold feet; irritable skin; worse at night on getting warm in bed, and from washing. Sulph. 3, 8h.

Protrusion and ready bleeding of haemorrhoids, constipation; moisture about anus, fissure; cramp and contraction of rectum. Phos. 6, 4h.

Great sensitiveness of the anus, itching, weakness of the sphincter and tendency to prolapse. Mur. ac 3x, 4h.

Soreness, itching, moisture; piles protrude, blue, suppurating and offensive; with burning; stitches in rectum Carb. v. 6, 4h.

Burning, itching at anus, excoriation; cutting pain after stool, protruding haemorrhoids, constipation; fissure. Nit ac. 6-30 4h.

Heat, rawness, soreness, loose motions, prolapse, bleeding; piles protrude like a bunch of grapes; constipation, or feeling of insecurity bowels Aloe 1, 4h.

Piles with burning and stinging in rectum; sore and smarting; mucous discharge; constipation Amm Mur 3x, 4h.

Piles burning as if pepper sprinkled on; tenesmus of rectum and bladder; tenacious mucus mixed with black blood; cutting colic before stool; tenesmus cutting and twisting during stool; after stool tenesmus, burning, thirst drinking causing shuddering, drawing pains in the back; piles swollen itching, throbbing; soreness in anus, bleeding or blue; with mucous discharge; with bloody mucous stools; with drawing pain in small of back and cutting in abdomen Caps 3, 4h.

Piles with constipation from inertia of the rectum, especially when connected with uterine disorders or pregnancy, piles bleed, but only with great pressure. Collin. ix – 3 4h.

Introduction: In this universe every effect has a cause. Sometimes the cause is latent and we know it from the effect; as is the case with roots which are hidden in the ground and only the sprouts or plants are seen above the ground. So every disease has a cause in some of our Karmas or previous actions behind them. If we remove the cause, there is no effect. Similarly if we remove the cause of a disease the effect is automatically removed. So our aim in curing an ailment should be to strike at the root-cause and not to combat against the effect. If we deal with the effect only as is the case with allopathic medicines, we only hold the disease in abeyance and it makes its head, at the earliest possible opportunity. So our aim should be to remove the cause.

Causes of the disease: Chief cause is the obstruction in the natural functions of the body. This body is a more ingenuous machine than all other machines invented by man. Let us take the case of a stove. If the pinhole is clogged or the pump is not in order, the stove does not work well and we have to remove the obstruction by pinning it. The fountain pen which is used by most of the persons nowadays, does not write well if it is not cleaned often and often. So also if we wish to keep our body or human machine in order we should remove obstructions if any from the alimentary canal so that it may work well and have good digestion and assimilation of the food we eat.

Want of Proper Exercise: Life means motion and stagnation is death. So like all other machines which do not work well, if they are not in use, this human machine does not work well if we do not have any kind of sufficient physical exercise in the form of hard bodily work or in its absence any kind of exercises. Bodily work or the exercises help in the right functioning of the physiological movement of the various organs of our body. Sedentary habits also are at the root of Piles and constipation which is chief cause of many diseases.

Checking of the urge to pass urine and stools and taking, strong purgatives: This kind of natural urge if it is not attended at the proper time, creates difficulties in the functions which are natural, puts pressure upon adjacent organs and creates heat and other disorders. Of course these effects are so slow that they cannot be procured at the very moment. So habits should be formed in such a way as not to interfere with the natural urge to pass stools.

Strong purgatives if resorted to in such a condition, goad the organs which are already in a diseased condition owing to obstruction, and create more harm than good to the delicate organs.

Wrong Feeding: Rottis prepared from white flour of mill ground wheat, boiled rice and Dal, prepared from mill pounded rice and mill pounded Dal, dried purees prepared from starch, create constipation, which ultimately leads to Piles. Too much eating of chillies and hot drinks also cause excessive heat in the body which leads to piles. Daily use of fried articles and high spiced vegetables, also causes piles.

Symptoms: Preliminary signs are heat in the anus, difficulty in passing stools, excrement consisting of clogs of faeces covered with streaks of blood. Piles are of the size of pea. They are caused by accumulated faecal matter pressing on the veins. If one overlooks the disease in the preliminary stage much blood passes through stools and there is intense pain in answering the calls of Nature. If much blood passes out, there is a feeling of exhaustion also.

Treatment: For quick cure, you should remove the causes. Only external application of medicines will not be much beneficial.

(1) Use enema daily for easy clearing of bowels.

(2) For healing piles inject juice of a lemon mixed with four times the quantity of water before going to bed or if lemon juice is not available inject only four ounces of water made cold in an earthenware pot.

(3) Live on fruits and milk for two weeks. Afterwards give up evening meal and instead use fruits and milk or vegetable or soup of vegetables available in the season.

(4) Take hip or sitz bath twice a day or at least put cold water pack or mud pack over the painful parts.

(5) Prolapsed piles may be inserted in their place.

(6) Ayurvedic Treatment: Take half a cup of juice of raddish leaves or leaves and roots with honey for taste, every morning.

(7) Apply lemon juice mixed with olive or ground nut or Til oil or inject this mixture.

(8) At night take one spoonful of Haritaki or Harad, i.e., myrobalan powder with water.

(9) Biochemic Remedies: Use daily in the morning Cal Phos 6x in the noon, Natrum Mur 6x and in the evening Cal Flour 6x.

(10) Piles need not be operated if they do not cause much trouble. Nature has the power to heal many diseases. But Nature's processes are slow and sure. Make a habit of answering the calls of nature at fixed hours. Try to do this daily whether you have the call for evacuation of bowels or not and after some time this good habit will be formed and you will have calls of nature at the proper time.

(11) Avoid sugar, rich food, spiced foods, sweetmeats, chillies and fatty foods.

(12) Hot water bath at night before going to bed, and

cold water in the morning are more invigorating to the nerves.

These remedies are within the reach of middle class men. Rich people can afford costly treatment of doctors. Poor people are not often sick as they have to work hard. Only the middle class men suffer much owing to their sedentary habits.

Nowadays diseases have a wide prevalence in our society. General vitality is very low. Reasons are too well-known to all. They are in want of proper food stuffs, milk and fruits and also dearness of all these articles. It is difficult for the Indian Government also to bring down prices of necessaries.

For the prevention of diseases and for better health amongst the young generation, rules for the maintenance of health must be taught compulsorily in schools. There should be constant examination of students, to nip diseases in the bud. Physical exercises should be made compulsory. Government is doing its best in this connection but co-operation of private bodies and guardians of students is also essential.

Everybody should become his own doctor. He should have at least one or two books on Health, Naturopathy and Biochemic Remedies.

Chapter XIX
DIVINE NAMAPATHY

When allopathy, homeopathy, chromopathy, naturo-pathy, Ayurvedapathy and all other pathies fail to cure a disease, the Divine Namapathy alone can save you. Name of the Lord is a sovereign specific, a sheet anchor, an infallible panacea and a cure-all for all diseases. It is an ideal or supreme "pick me up" in gloom and despair, depression and sorrow, in the daily battle of life or the struggle for existence.

There is a mysterious power in the Name. There is an inscrutable Sakti in God's name. All the divine potencies are hidden in Lord's name. It is a cream or quintessence of Chyavanprash, Makaradhwaja, almonds, Vasanta Kusumakar or Svarna Bhasma or gold oxide. It is a mysterious, ineffable divine injection '1910194'.

You can take this medicine of Nama Japa yourself for curing any disease. You can administer this marvellous medicine to other patients also in your house or elsewhere. Sit by the side of the patient and repeat the Name of the Lord with sincere devotion and faith like Hari Om, Sri Ram, Om Namassivaya, and sing His Names also *"Hare Rama Hare Rama Rama Rama Hare Hare – Hare Krishna Hare Krishna Krishna Krishna Hare Hare."* Pray for His mercy and grace. All maladies and agonies will come to an end. Do the treatment of Nama Japa for at least 2 hours in the morning and evening. You will find the miraculous effect within a short time. Both the doctor and the patient should have perfect faith in Lord's Name, His mercy and grace. The real doctor is only Lord Narayana:

Lord Dhanwantari, the physician of the three worlds (who expounded the Ayurvedic Medical science) has himself declared: "By the medicine of the repetition of Aychuta, Ananta, Govinda all diseases are cured.... this is my definite and honest declaration." In all treatments Lord Narayana is the real doctor. You find that even the world's best doctors fail to cure a dying king. You might have also heard of many instances where patients ailing from the worst type of diseases are cured miraculously where even the ablest doctors have declared the case hopeless. This itself is clear proof that there is Divine Hand behind all cures.

The Divine Name will eradicate the disease of birth and death and bestow on you. Moksha, liberation or Immortality.

The son of a landlord in Meerut was seriously ailing. Doctors pronounced the case to be absolutely hopeless. Bhaktas took the case in their hands. They did continuous Kirtan day and night for seven days around the bed of the patient. The patient stood up and began to sing God's name on the seventh day. He recovered completely. Such is the miraculous power of Sankirtan.

Chapter XX

MR. CONSTIPATION AND MRS. PILES

ACT I

(A tube-like cave-dwelling. The encircling wall is of cream-colour; artistic undulations on its surface impart life to it. It appears to throb with life as is indicated by the occasional wave-like movements on its surface. It has no doors on the sides; but there are openings above and below.

Over a hard black-and-brown clay stool is seated a monstrous figure, with a bottle of wine in one hand, and a dreadful poison in the other. His whole body is black and devilish. With his feet he is tightly closing the bottom opening of the room.

Occasionally yellowish clay-like substance dribbles through the aperture above; and this monstrous figure swallows portions of it with great gusto and on the rest of it he pours a little of the wine and a little of the poison, prepares a nice ball and sticks the ball on to the wall. As each ball is stuck thus to the wall the throbbing of the wall decreases. The wall grows a more and more 'dull'. The devil is obviously pleased with this phenomenon.)

The Devil: Ha! Ha! Ha! Ha! Thus should one strengthen his dwelling. (Gently taps the stool over which he is seated.) Stool! My dear stool! Harden up more and more. For, you form my seat here; you are dear to me even as my own life. You are my food, too! (Takes a pinch and eats.) How delicious! The older you grow, the greater is your nourishing power! My limbs get a special power. My feet are strengthened and I can more vigorously keep the hole at the bottom completely closed and thus ensure my happy livelihood here. Ha! Ha! Ha! Ha!

(Enter a demoness. She is red all over; red are her hair; red her lips; red her eyes; red her teeth. She holds a sharp dagger in her hands. She does not walk; but she dances forward. Every now and then she touches the wall with her dagger; and blood-like substance flows from the wall and escapes through the lower aperture. She is highly elated at this sight. She dances in ecstasy and kicks the wall with her feet.)

Demoness: Ha, ha, ha. Constipation, dear! When you invited me to live with, I did not expect such happiness, such comfort and such joy in your company. Indeed your house is a paradise for me. You are my dear, dear lord! (She embraces him.) We shall live together, for ever and ever. You are so valiant. You have great power. You are invincible. I am safe in your hand.

Constipation: Dearest, Piles! Ha, ha, ha. Well said. You are truly a wise woman; therefore, you have chosen me as your lord. Who can separate us? Who can put obstacles in the way of our enjoying each other? Look! I have build for us a lovely stool. The harder it grows, the more assured is our happiness. From the food that drops from above, I eat heartily. Don't think I am a glutton. I am a very prudent man. I have foresight. I mix this wine and this poison with the remnants of the food and stick it on the wall. My dearest, this cake produces auto-intoxication in Mr. Peristalsis, our arch-enemy who dwells in these walls. He is put for ever into deep slumber. I mix some poison also, so that Mr. Blood might grow blind and thus prevented from awakening Mr. Peristalsis.

Piles: My lord! You are indeed wise, too. Now that we

have become life-partners, tell me – who are your friends and who your enemies I shall not betray you; you may repose your fullest confidence in me.

Constipation: Why, my sweetheart! You ought to know since you are from today the mistress of my house. Listen. My only enemy is, of course, Mr. Peristalsis. If he regains his vigour, we are lost. But I have taken sufficient precautions to see that he sleeps more and more soundly. Ha, ha, ha, ha This poison extracted from the stool as it hardens, serves the purpose. My dear, do not let a worry cross thy brow. I have very devoted friends. The foremost of them who acts as my gate keeper is Mr. Palate. I have commanded him to itch, and to demand all sorts of wrong foods so that we shall always be provided with our own food. Mr. Palate is very efficient; he is very cunning also. He will demand food when our neighbour Mr. Stomach does not need it. Palate will despatch from above food in greater quantities than Mr. Stomach needs. This is all part of my diplomacy, my dear, so that I could get what I need without fail.

Piles: Is Stomach your friend or enemy?

Constipation: If Mr. Palate is indifferent in his job, and if Mr. Stomach as a consequence gets only as much food as he himself needs, naturally he absorbs everything in entirety and throws down only that which we shall also have to discard. And, when Mr. Stomach does his work properly, then Mr. Peristalsis will also get his strength, will be awakened and will cooperate with Mr. Stomach in throwing right away the rubbish from Mr. Stomach's house. Then, naturally Mr. Stomach becomes our enemy.

If, on the other hand, Mr. Palate is vigilant and overloads Mr. Stomach, the latter gets tired, overburdened with work; and he neglects even his normal function! Then he seeks our friendship.

Piles: God be thanked; for we have a very good friend in Mr. Palate. Let us pray that he shall ever be vigilant. We shall then live for ever together.

ACT II

(Constipation's bungalow. Constipation is happily seated on his hardened stool.)

Piles rushes into the room from the opening above.

Piles: My Lord! We are done for. A great enemy is approaching. His attendants are shouting at the top of their voice: 'His Exalted Highness Maharajadhiraja Castor Oil is coming. Leave the way!' They are coming with great speed. Oh, what a calamity. What shall we do now? They threaten to seep everything away.

Constipation: My dearest! Fear not.

Fear not. I shall soon devise some plan. Do you recollect that some time ago we had a threat from Mr. Tea and Mr. Coffee. Do you remember how quickly I made friendship with them? Now they do not affect us. After temporarily depriving us of our food, they have surrendered themselves to us. We have made an alliance with them.

Piles (interrupting): My Lord! this enemy is of a different nature altogether. He is very destructive. What shall we do? Please think of a way out.

Constipation: Fear not. I shall not be vanquished. I am not a child to be defeated by Mr. Castor Oil. (Thinks) Once he very nearly killed me; by Lord's grace I escaped. We should not fight with him face to face. We should adapt a cunning method. We should recede to the walls. Even at the cost of our food the stool, which will inevitably be swept away, we should protect ourselves. Come; stick to the walls. Let Castor Oil pass off.

(They both cling to the wall. With great noise and tumultuous uproar, Castor Oil comes from the aperture above. The attendants pull down Constipation's stool and wash it away through the opening at the bottom).

(After Castor Oil had left, Constipation and Piles move away from the wall. Constipation looks paler.)

Constipation: (weeping) Oh, my stool has been swept away. Our food has gone! What shall we do now? (Suddenly brightens up.) By my diplomacy I have saved our lives. Food will come again. We shall grow fat again. My dearest! Worry not.

Piles: Dear Constipation! All the time I was watching our worst enemy, Peristalsis. I found that Mr. Castor Oil did nothing to awaken him; but Mr. Castor Oil merely passed along! Then I was sure we are safe.

Constipation: You are right, dear Piles. And, I have telegraphically commanded Mr. Palate to carry on his work more vigorously. Castor Oil temporarily overwhelms him; this naturally produces a serious reaction; as soon as Castor Oil has passed away, Mr. Palate will be even more brisk in his itching and demand for more and more food. Bravo! We shall be happy again.

(Food begins to dribble through the aperture above; Constipation swallows it, prepares the stool with it and also prepares the paste for the wall. The lower aperture is closed again. Thus Constipation and Piles live happily on.)

ACT III
Scene I

(A Dining Hall. Around the dinner table are seated a number of physicians, belonging to various systems of medicine. A Conference over Constipation is in progress.)

Dr. Roy: Gentlemen, constipation does not at all worry us, allopaths. We have quite a number of purgatives, strong and mild and we can always deal with constipation without any difficulty at all. In fact, it is not a disease that need be treated by a doctor; even an ordinary compounder will dispense the medicines, and if the patient is a little educated, he can himself get the pills — castophene, brooklax etc., direct from the shop and take them. Where piles are also found, then, I advise surgical operation to get them removed. This, too, is very, very simple nowadays. At the same time, we give Vitamin B complex injections and give also good general tonics to tone the patient up and restore vigour to his digestive organs.

Dr. Achintyanand: Friends, we Homeopaths understand that constipation may lead to serious complications and might poison the system. We have in our therapeutics quite a number of remedies which will completely eradicate constipation. It requires an intelligent handling, no doubt and each case to be studied on its own merits and careful individualisation made before prescribing the most appropriate remedy. I have myself cured many serious cases of constipation and piles; and I am confident that without the least surgical interference, both these diseases can be permanently cured.

Vaidyaraj Satchidanand: Brothers, to those suffering from constipation I advise the regular use of Triphala. In Ayurveda, too, we have excellent remedies for both constipation and piles. Sometimes, *isaphgul* also helps. The chewing of myrobalan relieves constipation.

Sri Hariom: When all is said and done, it is naturopathy that really effects the cure. None of your medicines will work if the patient does not observe dietetic restrictions. He should give up taking tea and coffee in excesses. Taking a glass of water the first thing in the morning, with the juice of a lemon, a spoonful of honey and a pinch of salt dissolved in it, is wonderful. A little brisk walk and a few simple abdominal exercises will tone the muscles of the abdomen and increase peristalsis. When the case is acute, however, enema is inevitable; but this is absolutely harmless.

Yogiraj Vishnu: I have taught Asanas and Pranayama to hundreds of students and have never suffered from constipation or piles. Even those who were suffering from these diseases previously have been completely cured. Halasana, Paschimottanasana, Salabhasana and Sirshasana (which cures constipation caused by intra-abdominal pressure); Agnisara and Nauli Kriya—all these wonderfully tone up the abdominal muscles and ensure peristalsis. Maha-Mudra, in addition to these, cures piles, too.

Sevananda: Sirs, here I have brought a patient who suffers from both constipation and piles. Many remedies have been tried by him; and most of them relieve him temporarily, but the trouble invariably returns. Just as the wise aspirant adopts the combined method in order to win a victory over his mind, just as the Yoga of Synthesis is practised in order to attain Self-realisation quickly, even so I suggest that a combined attack is made on this constipation and piles, so that the victory is assured.

All Doctors: Hear, hear. We all agree.

Sevananda: Let Sri Hariom supervise the patient's diet, and Vishnu teach him Asanas and Kriyas; Vaidyaraj may relieve the acute disease by giving a strong purgative, and if the trouble returns, Roy can give a pill or two to ease the situation. In the meantime, the Homeopath might select the best remedy to bring about complete recovery. If, after some time, we feel it necessary, we shall get the piles removed by operation.

(All Doctors agree)   (Curtain)

Scene II

(Constipation's bungalow. Constipation and piles are in great distress.)

Constipation: I am utterly.defeated. I have no place to stand. I am not given the least opportunity to gather strength. Against this relentless persecution I am unable to stand. Peristalsis also awakened. Oh, I am dying. I am gone.

Piles: O Lord, when you are gone, how shall I live? I too shall follow thee.